HOMOEOPATHIC SKETCHES OF CHILDREN'S TYPES

OTHER BOOKS BY CATHERINE R. COULTER:

Portraits of Homoeopathic Medicines. 3 vols.
(Vol. 3 includes "Portrait of Indifference")

Vol. 1 ISBN: 0971308217
Vol. 2 ISBN: 0971308225
Vol. 2 ISBN: 0971308233

Nature and Human Personality:
Homoeopathic Archetypes
ISBN: 0971308241

A Homoeopathic Approach to Cancer
(co-authored with Dr. A.U. Ramakrishnan)
ISBN: 0971308209

✦

All books available from Ninth House Publishing
Telephone: 1-800-336-1695 • www.homeopathyworks.com

HOMOEOPATHIC SKETCHES OF CHILDREN'S TYPES

Catherine R. Coulter

Ninth House Publishing

BERKELEY SPRINGS, WEST VIRGINIA

2001

This book consists, for the most part, of selected passages adapted by
Catherine R. Coulter from her previously published works,
Portraits of Homoeopathic Medicines, vols. 1, 2, and 3.
These books are available from Ninth House Publishing.

EDITOR	Marian Coulter
PRODUCTION	Barbara Shaw
COVER DESIGN	Diane Beasley
ILLUSTRATIONS AND COVER ILLUSTRATION	Erin O'Connor

Printed in the United States of America
by McNaughton & Gunn, Inc.
Third Printing

Published by Ninth House Publishing
260 J R Hawvermale Way
Berkeley Springs, West Virginia 25411
Telephone: 1-800-336-1695
Web site: www.homeopathyworks.com

LIBRARY OF CONGRESS CATALOGING IN PUBLICATION DATA

Coulter, Catherine R.
Homoeopathic Sketches of Children's Types
Includes suggested readings and index
ISBN 0-9713082-6-8
1. Homoeopathy–Materia medica and therapeutics.
2. Typology. 3. Medicine. 4. Psychology

2001118229

Aude Sapere
(Dare to Try)

EPIGRAPH TO SAMUEL HAHNEMANN'S
Organon of Medicine

Acknowledgments

My daughter, Marian Coulter, has lent to this book her invaluable editorial assistance; and Mary Yano was ever generous with her time, support, and thoughtful advice throughout the typing of the manuscript. To both these true friends the author extends her heartfelt gratitude.

An additional thanks is owed to Suzanne Wakefield for her excellent editorial suggestions.

Contents

Introduction

The growing child, as he or she evolves toward maturity, passes through a series of stages of development, each one of which presents its own particular set of challenges that must be confronted. These archetypal stages of growth and learning are mirrored in the homoeopathic remedies, which are used to assist the child to take in stride the ofttimes difficult passages from youth to adulthood.*

The science of homoeopathy, founded by Samuel Hahnemann around the beginning of the nineteenth century, is based on the Law of Similars. In other words, a medicinal substance capable of producing a set of morbid symptoms in the healthy individual will remove similar symptoms occurring in an ailing individual. From this basic tenet there evolves a set of assumptions about illness, health, and healing that are pivotal to the homoeopathic method and approach.

The overriding assumption is the belief in a "vital force"— an innate energy in all things living that is always striving for

---

* *Homoeopathic Sketches of Children's Types* is a companion volume to *Nature and Human Personality: Homoeopathic Archetypes,* in which adult types are analyzed and described. Like their adult counterparts, these children's archetypes are, for the most part, adaptations of the author's *Portraits of Homoeopathic Medicines: Psychophysical Analyses of Selected Constitutional Types,* vols. 1-3 (see Suggested Readings).

harmony and balance. Symptoms are signs of the body's efforts to heal itself, and the homoeopathic remedies, in their "similarity" to a patient's symptoms, support the self-healing efforts of the vital force.

The second important assumption, and one on which all homoeopathic prescribing is based, is of the "wholeness" of the individual. In a truly holistic approach, homoeopathy recognizes that physical illnesses have a mental-emotional aspect, while mental-emotional illnesses have a physical aspect. In the process of prescribing for the child's healthy growth and promoting his (or her) well-being, the practitioner always takes into consideration both categories of symptoms, as viewed in their dynamic interaction.

This method of addressing a medicine to the totality of a patient's symptoms is called "constitutional prescribing," and the medicinal substance that embraces not only the sum total of a patient's physical, mental, and emotional symptoms, but his personality picture as well, is called the "constitutional remedy." Thus a child is said to be a *Sulphur* or a *Lycopodium,* a *Pulsatilla* or a *Natrum muriaticum,* depending on the medicinal substance that best fits his outward appearance, temperament, and disposition, according to how he behaves in sickness and in health and how he responds to difficulties or happy occasions. His type is also indicated by his gestures, manner, voice, his hopes and fears, likes and dislikes, strengths and weaknesses, or his particular talents. All these traits help determine the constitutional remedy—although, certainly, a child (according to circumstances or temperament) might be an alloy of two or three types, around which he will gravitate during his early years.

And because there is bound to be overlap between the different types, they will, on occasion, be compared and contrasted.*

The homoeopathic typology is, to be sure, directed primarily toward healing, and the remedies presented in this book are the ones most frequently prescribed "constitutionally" in pediatric practice (the two exceptions being *Belladonna* and *Chamomilla,* which are usually prescribed for some *specific* or *acute* ailment). But there is another aspect to these archetypes: with the recognition of types comes superior understanding, and with superior understanding comes the ability to better guide and assist a child to achieve his fullest potential.

---

* In these pages the remedies have been paired off because of a certain physical or emotional kinship in their healthy or disruptive energies. However, there is in constitutional prescribing a clear hierarchy of the remedies, and in certain pairs the first will be employed far more often than the second. In these instances the dominant remedy is marked with a section mark (§).

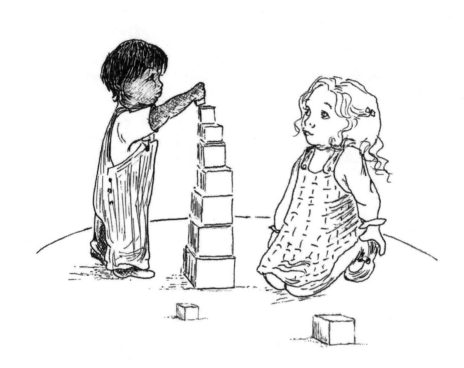

Calcarea carbonica §

(CARBONATE OF LIME, TAKEN FROM THE MIDDLE LAYER OF THE OYSTER SHELL)

C *alcarea carbonica* is the infant's and young child's constitutional remedy *par excellence*: it plays a significant role in the assimilation of calcium and other nutrients and thereby helps to promote the healthy development of nerves, glands, skin, teeth, and bones. In the early years of tremendous growth, many a youngster will start out in life as a *Calcarea carbonica* before he develops (according to environment, heredity, or chance circumstances) into some other constitutional type.*

In outward appearance the typical *Calcarea carbonica* baby is soft and flabby, with a big head that perspires profusely (especially at night in bed, during sleep), often emitting a sourish or cheesy odor. The potbellied toddler looks healthy and well-fed but is not as robust as he appears to be, and he tends to

---

§ See footnote in Introduction, page xi.

*For stylistic purposes, the masculine gender has been employed throughout this book to denote both sexes, except when otherwise stated.

operate in low gear. This can be observed in such symptoms as delayed closure of the fontanelles, lingering cradle cap, difficult or delayed dentition, and slowness in learning to walk or some other basic motor skill. Often the metabolism is slow and the circulation poor; the child is chilly despite being well-covered. He may be clumsy in his movements and lack physical endurance. Even slight exertion fatigues him, and he might suffer from car-, sea-, or airsickness, as if rapid movement in a vehicle were tantamount to physical effort. At times, too, *Calcarea carbonica* is slow in beginning to talk. The knowledge is there— the words just waiting to be brought out—but he refuses to be *hurried* into talking, with the result that one day the previously inarticulate child will suddenly express himself with surprising maturity.

An example was the two-year-old, not yet talking, who wanted to attract her resting mother's attention. Being of a considerate disposition, she came up and leaned her head against her mother's bed and softly whispered, "Mommy?" No response. She then changed her tone to a still whispered but more imperious, "Mom-my!" Still no response. She then tried the more formal, "Mother?" Her mother pretended to sleep on, hoping the child would leave, but instead of leaving, there was a long pause. Then the child tried her mother's nickname, "Becky?" The silence continued, followed by the next query, "Rebecca?" Since her mother kept her eyes closed, she next resorted to the Spanish housekeeper's form of address, "Señora!" Another pause, and finally in a desperate last resort, "Mrs. N___, *please!*" At which point the vanquished mother had to concede.

Thus, it is not unusual for the *Calcarea carbonica* child to hit on an imaginative and original method of resolving his difficulties. Although one would never describe this type as "the sharpest knife in the drawer," in fact, that which appears to be slowness is often the phlegmatic child's tendency to operate less on a logical, linear plane than on the more circuitous level of feelings and sensitivities. For instance, listening to a nursery school lesson on whales, a *Sulphur* or *Arsenicum* child will absorb the fascinating details of their enormous size, strength, and food consumption, and later relay them to others. A *Calcarea* child will also listen wide-eyed and attentive to the information, but later that night, cowering in his or her mother's lap, might remark in an awed tone, "Mommy, I think there must be whales in the dark!" Similarly, the young child who resides on a main street in a city or town, if asked where he lives, might reply, "Just walk straight, straight along the big road till you reach a pretty house at the end. There's a canary there in the dining room who chirps all day because he's happy."

Typically, the *Calcarea carbonica* child is even-tempered, nonaggressive, not unduly demanding. The infant is content to stay where he is put, curiously inspecting his fingers or toes or quietly playing with a toy, turning it over as he examines it from all angles. Or he sits or lies quietly, staring intently at one person or fixedly at some object, or just calmly looking around. The toddler goes his own way, imperturbably climbing over furniture or the knees of adults as he explores his surroundings. When permitted to roam on his own, he responds to obstacles in a very particular way: instead of demanding adult help, he will push, grunt, pull, strain as he tries to get around or dislodge them. It is heartening to watch him resolve difficulties by himself instead of complaining or crying. But by the same token, because of his independence, the child, although friendly, is intrinsically less tractable, less eager to please than *Phosphorus* or *Pulsatilla*. Placid he may be, but he undoubtedly has a mind of his own.

There does exist a shadow side, however, to the disposition of this fundamentally calm, contented, endearing youngster: the ungovernable temper tantrums that arise from no discernible provocation. If one cause is removed, he finds another to scream about and, once started, he is nearly impossible to quiet. In counteracting a young child's tendency to tantrums, this remedy has few equals. But as noted earlier, since the *Calcarea* disposition is generally placid and even-tempered, often the child does not want to throw tantrums to get his own way. What then is his principal defense against the stronger forces that surround and govern him, imposing their will on his?

The answer is obstinacy. *Calcarea carbonica* is among the most obstinate, if not *the* most obstinate, of constitutional types. "No! No! No! I won't! I won't! I won't! You can't make me!" he cries, mulishly digging in his heels; or he silently refuses to budge, and nothing short of sheer physical force can induce him to capitulate. He can therefore be harder to influence than the most actively rebelling *Sulphur,* unruly *Tuberculinum,* or obdurate *Nux vomica* (who, however, comes a close second for obstinacy). Once *Calcarea* discovers the efficacy of stubborn resistance, he clings to this tactic with tenacity.

In the young child, this stubbornness often manifests at mealtimes. No amount of pressure can force him to eat what he does not want to. Not only is the appetite capricious but, even more, it is restricted. In contrast to *Sulphur's* liking for strong-tasting, unusual, and varied foods, *Calcarea* is a picky eater, with tastes running to the bland and the monotonous. He might have only one or two acceptable dishes. One child will only eat a hot dog on half a roll one day, alternating with a hamburger on half a bun the next; another will only eat cheese or peanut butter and jelly sandwiches; a third will only eat pasta or potatoes; a fourth will only drink milk and hardly touch anything else. Yet even while eating small amounts of extremely limited foods, he still remains plump. Generally speaking, however, and as he grows older, the child becomes greatly interested in food. He loves to eat—especially starchy, creamy, and dairy foods (although the last may not be well tolerated), and bland ones (for instance, he likes his pizza without pepperoni).

If pressured in school, *Calcarea carbonica* puts up a passive resistance. Other types fight authority; *Calcarea* balks. Thus, if the child is not responding well in school, it may be that the environment is too pressured or the teacher too pushy. When one *Calcarea* three-year-old was asked to explain his obstinate, uncooperative behavior in nursery school, he answered simply, "It's because of my teacher. She makes me ner-vi-ous." Indeed, she was an intense, driving type, ill-suited to the unhurried, independent, little boy.

Sometimes, the child is well-adjusted socially, but the learning process exerts no appeal. He fears being ridiculed for slowness, easily feels overwhelmed, and hence is incapable of performing at all; or conversely, he might conscientiously try to keep up with the rest of the class, yet real success eludes him. If he does succeed, it is by spending a disproportionate amount of time on his work, with the head literally becoming heated from mental exertion. And a not uncommon physical manifestation of the type's resistance to academic pressures is a child's inexplicable stomachaches that come on just before or toward the end of the school day.

Contributing to the *Calcarea* picture of resistance to pressure of any kind is an inherent indolence. For instance, much prodding might be required to get the child to start on his homework, and then he may lack the mental stamina to follow through to the finish. On the other hand, once his interest has been captured, even the fundamentally indolent youngster might not be able to tear himself away. In mental pursuits he finds it difficult to pace himself. There is the initial stubborn resistance to be overcome, but once enthralled, he knows no moderation. Nor is the type bored or fatigued by repetition. He will (if interested) go over the same material again and again. And the young *Calcarea carbonica* never tires of being told or read the same story, night after night, and corrects the narrator if he deviates by so much as one word from the original version.

At the same time as he needs to go about things in his own way, the *Calcarea* youngster requires the security of a structured environment in which to develop. He is not the type to thrive on his own but needs a delicate balance of structure and freedom to accommodate his plodding, *sui generis* style and to encourage his healthy growth. From time to time, the child himself recognizes this need for structure and discipline and will, surprisingly, impose it on himself. One three-year-old with a poor appetite was eventually sent to stand in the corner until he agreed to eat at least a minimal amount of his meals. Henceforth, whenever he felt resistant, he would get up from the table and say, "I want into the corner," and proceed to place himself there until he was ready to come back and eat. Or a nine-year-old, when left unpunished for a misdemeanor, solemnly instructed his parents, "You send me to my room and make me stay there *long*—on bread and water. I was bad and shouldn't get away with things like this." Another slightly older *Calcarea* boy who usually ate desserts and candy in large quantities decided to give them up for Lent, just to see if he *could* do it. When Lent was over, he announced that the discipline was good for him and that he intended to undergo the same regimen the following year. And a *Calcarea,* a fourteen-year-old girl, who wrote poetry in highly structured verse forms for her English class assignments because blank verse was "too easy," was likewise voluntarily subjecting herself to a strict discipline.

The *Calcarea* nature is a sensitive and vulnerable one, as reflected in a variety of fears and anxieties. The child is afraid of the dark, of going upstairs to bed by himself. He wakes up screaming from night terrors, imagines monsters under his bed, or sees horrifying faces and frightening creatures in the dark. Sometimes he exhibits a highly specific phobia. One child will be afraid of spiders, and spiders only; another of ants; a third of caterpillars; a fourth of mice. The fear is not of insects, rodents, or reptiles in general (although this more general fear is also possible), but a seemingly irrational fear of one particular species. A youngster will fearlessly walk up to the biggest dog or reach out to pat an elephant in the zoo, will stoically confront snakes and rats, but will exhibit such an aversion to some innocuous bug as to be panicked even by a replica of one. One little girl insisted that her parents cut the ladybug buttons off her bathrobe and remove a ladybug appliqué from the pocket of a dress because they were giving her nightmares.

Another inordinate fear of the young child is being away from home. An extreme example was a two-month-old baby, a contented and placid child who, from the day she was born, hardly ever cried. But when taken on her first weekend visit to friends, she took one look at the unfamiliar surroundings and broke out in such uncontrollable screaming that the parents had to take her home. The wise and experienced attributed the incident to coincidence or, perhaps, fear of something in the new house. No baby of two months, they claimed, could realize she was away from home. But two weeks later, when the mother tried to leave her at the house of a sitter, the same scene was repeated. She was howling inconsolably even before her mother had left the room; yet at home she was fine with any sitter. Likewise, even the older child might feel anxious sleeping over at a friend's house, and might ask to go home.

The child is slow to recover from shock, and the effect of a frightening experience can be felt for years. One three-year-old boy's history of petit mal seizures began with the sight of a snake swallowing a frog. Another youngster, thrown into near convulsions when a mouse jumped out at her from a drawer, remained subject to longlasting twitchings and spasms whenever she was frightened, until *Calcarea carbonica* cured her. Frightening impressions received from television, from a book, or something simply overheard in conversation might give him nightmares and haunt him night and day. An older child will accept a lower grade in school rather than read a book that describes violence or harsh treatment of children or animals.

The type can similarly be sensitive to the small upsetting incidents of everyday life. He cannot understand what motivates others to behave irrationally or to be gratuitously mean. Nor need their behavior affect him personally. He is terribly upset that Susie did not invite Sarah to her birthday party or that Jessie, who used to be friends with Eric, was nasty to him today.

He is more upset by these trifling fallings-out in the endless feuds of children than are the principals themselves. Jessie and Eric will eventually make up or go on to other things, but *Calcarea* is left behind to worry about the harsh ways of this world. These are the Charlie Browns of the world; lovable but naïve—often the last to "catch on" and never quite able to keep up with the life that whizzes past them. In one *Peanuts* sequence, Charlie Brown stares in bewilderment at the frenetic activity of the children's world around him and laments, "I never know what's going on!"

Sensitivity to criticism is another aspect of this type's vulnerability. To the teacher or parent he might seem to take criticism well, but at a deeper level he is affected by it. He is not immediately devastated, nor does he burst into argument, self-justifications, or tears of indignation; he is slow to react. Rather, he withdraws into himself, bruised and silent, and refuses in the future to try. Many an adult *Calcarea*'s lack of initiative or fear of failure stems directly from such early childhood criticism, which a more hardy constitutional type would simply ignore.

For some children, then, *Calcarea carbonica,* the remedy, acts as a protective shield against the harshness of the world, while for others it acts as the irritant that nudges them out of their fears and sensitivities (like that irritating grain of sand that stimulates the oyster to form a pearl), the better to prepare them for the challenges of adulthood. In either case, the remedy plays a vital role in fortifying a child's psyche—as well as in strengthening his muscles, nerves and bones.

۲۶

The physical symptoms calling for *Calcarea carbonica* in

children are myriad. Following is merely a thumbnail sketch.

There is a tendency to swollen tonsils and enlarged adenoids, cervical, submandibular, and other glands; to an unending series of colds, earaches, and attacks of bronchitis during winter months. Chronic snuffles or a runny nose are caused by narrowness of the nasal passages or by the poor assimilation of dairy products. Thus, a poor digestion is often encountered, as seen by an infant's easy vomiting and a tendency to spit up even mother's milk, bouts of diarrhea or a pale stool (as if lacking bile pigment), or constipation. Idiosyncratically, the child can be constipated for days on end without any seeming discomfort.

The modalities encountered are: *worse* from cold in every form; from exertion of every form (physical, mental, eyestrain, ascending stairs); during dentition; from pressure of tight clothes; from milk and eggs (which, however, the child might crave); or during the full moon; *better* from warmth of every form (air, clothes, food); being allowed to proceed in his own way and at his own pace.

Belladonna

(DEADLY NIGHTSHADE)

There is one additional feature of *Calcarea carbonica* that is essential to note: it has an "acute" counterpart in *Belladonna*—a remedy that is frequently needed in a variety of children's common ailments. In other words, when a child is repeatedly subject to carsickness or airsickness, ear infections, sore or strep throats, swollen glands, rheumatic pains, boils, or high fevers, which respond well at the time to *Belladonna,* then *Calcarea carbonica,* prescribed "constitutionally," will often prevent recurrences of these acute ailments.

Whatever the specific physical condition, the *Belladonna* picture is often one of cerebral excitation, with extreme restlessness, twitchings, startings, convulsive movements, and fibrillations; all symptoms characterized by the suddenness of their onset or the violence of the attack. The child is extremely sensitive to light, to the slightest noise, pressure or jar, and to drafts. He cannot lie down flat (he is better when propped up by pillows) or lie still, but rocks in bed and moans or thrashes about. The nature of his pain is throbbing or cramping, with much burning, whether of the eye, throat, head, or chest; and usually bright redness accompanies any infection or inflammation. During fevers, the mental state is one of pronounced agitation and turmoil, at times reaching the point of delirium and hallucinations. The child screams, rages, and strikes. He sees frightening monsters and hideous faces; or he evinces a desire to escape from something pursuing him. Physically, the face is bright red, sometimes one-sided or with one cheek redder than the other, and the pupils are widely dilated. The whole body can be heated, although frequently one hand or foot is hotter than the other or the extremities are cooler than the rest of the body.

A key symptom is the pain comes in waves: commencing (the child begins to show signs of restlessness and discomfort), crescendoing (he starts moaning and thrashing about), reaching a peak (he cries out in pain), then decrescendoing (gradually the attack or spasm subsides). After that, the child is quiet until the next wave of pain or discomfort, which recurs at regular intervals.

Finally, *Belladonna* has a corresponding wave-like pattern in its time modality. Pains begin in the afternoon (between 3:00 and 6:00 p.m.), crescendo at night (especially between 9:00 p.m. and 3:00 a.m.), and subside by early morning. Then a period of relative comfort follows until the mid or late afternoon.

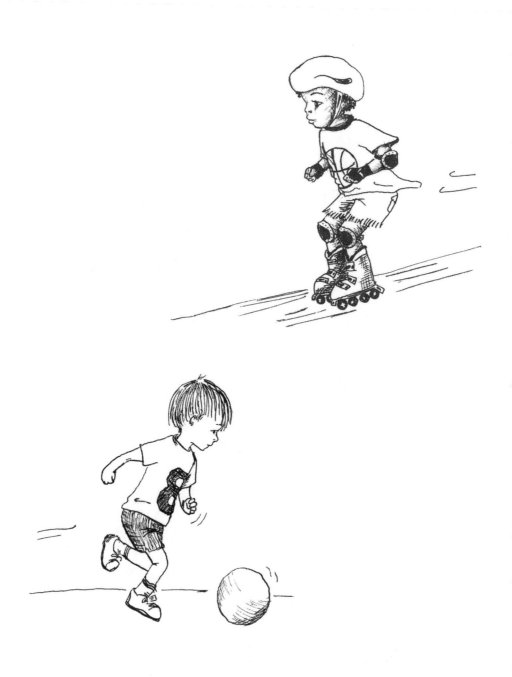

Sulphur§

(SUBLIMATED SULPHUR—THE ELEMENT)

S *ulphur* is unquestionably another one of the sovereign remedies in the homoeopathic treatment of children. Every child, at some stage in his development between infancy and adolescence, can profit from this remedy's versatile healing powers. And yet, though commanding a wide range of childhood symptoms and characteristics, a definite archetypal picture of *Sulphur* emerges strong and clear for all to recognize.

The child is usually warm-blooded—uncomfortable in warm weather, a warm room (he wants the windows open), taking warm baths, or wearing warm clothing. Even in cold weather he dons only a sweater and trousers, ignoring hat, gloves, and jacket. Parents must constantly struggle with him over wearing a coat. He wriggles and resists, arguing that he does not need one, and defines a sweater as "something you have to wear when your mother is cold." He tends to perspire freely, his extremities are warm, with hot or sweaty palms, and the ears are often red. Additionally, he might complain of burning in any part of the body. For instance, during the day he likes to run

15

around barefoot because his feet burn when he has shoes on, and in bed at night he kicks off the blankets to expose his burning soles. He so likes the feel of cold air on his hot head that even in winter he sleeps with the windows open. And an infant's skin rashes are often burning hot.

The theme of heat carries over into the realm of food preferences. For the most part, the *Sulphur* child has a healthy appetite; he likes most foods, including ethnic, hot, and spicy dishes. One of his preferred foods is pizza *with* pepperoni, while his most typical aversion (because of the blandness) is cooked vegetables—specifically broccoli, Brussels sprouts, spinach, and lima beans. The type also displays significant thirst for cold drinks: milk (which, however, might disagree with him), juices, and especially iced carbonated drinks, which he downs in large gulps, as if to cool his overheated body.

Likewise, in behavior, *Sulphur* frequently presents a picture of heat: the infant is restless, active, hard to quiet, and continually on the go, fussing against whatever holds him down or holds him still. The toddler hates being washed, dressed, put to bed, or seated at a table. He may literally have to be tied to his chair to be kept sitting through a meal. As the child grows older, rowdiness and noise-making become intrinsic to his nature: slamming doors, banging on things, barreling down the stairs, loud shouting, and generally making noise for its own sake. Adults are constantly telling him, "Keep quiet! Be still! Sit down!" "Stop it! *Whatever* you're doing—stop it!"

But, in contrast to the *Calcarea Carbonica* child who tends to be an observer, *Sulphur* is a "doer" and needs to be active. In school he cannot sit quietly, but fidgets at his desk, speaks out of turn, and constantly jumps up to go to the bathroom, get a drink of water, or for whatever other excuse he can think of. He is not only energetic but also inherently creative—initiating projects, embarking on new ventures, and refusing to allow life to become stagnant. In fact, he feels it to be his particular obligation to keep people and events on the move.* Some boys must always be talking. If they have nothing particular to say, they will babble or talk nonsense in order to fill the unendurable silence or to attract attention. Often they are quiet only when listening to music. Even here, however, the music must be stimulating, and the youngster plays it at a volume that deafens others but bothers him not at all. He may later join a school band or orchestra, or an informal jazz or rock band, because he enjoys making music in a group—the louder the better.

The disposition tends to be fiery, eruptive, and pugnacious. The boy flushes scarlet, yells, and stomps in anger or displeasure. But the reason for the display of temper is easily detectable and, once removed, the flare-up subsides as rapidly as it came on. The bad mood vanishes, the incident is forgotten, and two minutes later he is back to normal. In fact, the youngster's best friend might well be a fellow *Sulphur* with whom he quarrels and makes up interminably, at times engaging in an exhilarating fistfight.

Yet, although the type can be demanding, assertive, and quick-tempered, and the rowdiness can reach the level of the terrorizing youngster in O. Henry's short story *The Ransom of Red Chief* (in which the boy's kidnappers are willing to pay his father money to take him back), the nature is basically sunny

---

* Although the archetypal picture that follows is encountered more frequently in boys, naturally it can apply to girls also.

and optimistic, often remarkably uncomplaining, and possessing the buoyant outlook of those two charming *Sulphur* immortals, Tom Sawyer and Dennis the Menace. The boy emanates heat, but like fire he also radiates cheerfulness.

From an early age *Sulphur* is convinced that he knows best and fights to be left alone to try. "By myself! By myself!" the young child cries, as he struggles to tie his shoelaces or attempts some other difficult task. And the older child insists on doing it "My way!" In any sphere of life, given the slightest opportunity, he grabs hold of the ball and runs off with it, making up his own rules as he goes along and expecting others to follow. This aggressive unwillingness to cooperate with the group or social rules is often attributed to selfishness, but in actuality it is generated more by extreme independence and resentment of any outside interference. And time, only, can alter this trait.

The lively boy might turn his energies to becoming a disruptive influence in the home or at school. It is not that he is scheming or underhanded. Scorning dissimulation, *Sulphur* is usually open and straightforward, even in his mischievous or negative behavior. He disrupts by causing a commotion, or by being overly boisterous and a showoff. Continually striving for effect, he will brag loudly of his real or imagined "macho" feats, even if they are unruly ones. One way or another, he is determined to be noticed.

On the other hand, the boy who is the social core of the class is also frequently a *Sulphur*. He is still making waves, still asserting himself, still seeking recognition, but in a more constructive way. Manifesting undeniable leadership skills, he energetically organizes group activities in which all must participate. Indeed, because he is constantly generating big and bold ideas, he needs others to carry them out and surrounds himself with those willing to do so—while he, himself, is already onto his next grandiose scheme.

Sulphur can possess a strong materialistic streak. Even the young child can be quite ferocious in grabbing a toy away from another. "Gimme it! Hey, I want that ball! It's mine!" are among his earliest phrases, and all the while he resolutely protects his own: "Hey, that's *my* truck. Don't touch it!" The type was recognized in the eighteen-month-old boy who, sitting on his mother's knee, was tugging at her earrings, shouting, "Mine! Mine!" with a determined expression on his little face.

As the boy grows older the materialist in him begins to collect things: rocks, shells, old locks and keys, baseball cards. He even collects broken toys fished out of trash cans—whatever catches his fancy, regardless of its worth. The *Sulphur* girl is more selective: she collects dolls or stuffed animals or tiny china knickknacks, which she crowds onto her shelves where she can see them all. Then she spends hours sorting, arranging, and rearranging these pretty objects. The boy, on the other hand, who hates to pick up, is more likely to shove his collection into a drawer or leave it in a pile on the floor. The salient point here is that *Sulphur*, the packrat, is constitutionally unable to throw things away and hates to part with objects, however useless. One thirteen-year-old girl, ordered to discard some of the books and toys she had outgrown, wailed piteously, "How can you expect me to get rid of them when I can't even bear to throw away my fourth grade spelling tests!"

No matter how cluttered his room is, *Sulphur* knows exactly where everything is and cannot stand having anything moved or removed. He must be able, at any moment, to lay his hands on some particular object and dislikes anything to be out of his sight or reach. One three-year-old walked around with five (not one, but *five*) pacifiers in his possession, tied onto a string: one in his mouth, one tightly clenched in each fist, and the remaining two dangling from each arm where he could see them. If any of the five disappeared, he would fly into a passion. After receiving *Sulphur* for a physical complaint, he one day came to his parents and said, "I think, in fact, I'm getting too old for my pacifiers. I'm going to give them *all* away to Santa Claus. D'you think he'll come in the summer [it was July] to get 'em?" However, being a true *Sulphur* type, he requested an electric train in exchange for his well-chewed pacifiers.

During his boyhood stage *Sulphur* loves swapping goods, and seldom does he emerge the loser in these transactions. Although, here again, the reverse can be encountered and he will happily trade a good camera or brand new penknife for an irresistible sack of worthless old toys—and be extremely pleased with himself. This also is the boy who is completely satisfied with the frayed soccer ball and rickety old bicycle that he has owned for years and wishes for nothing more. Interestingly, the extremes of materialism and antimaterialism meet in this type.

As do the extremes of selfishness and unselfishness. For instance, in his strong attachment to his possessions, *Sulphur* may be unwilling to share them and, if urged to do so, will hang onto them for dear life. He might even resent lending out an impersonal and easily replaceable object, such as a stapler or a pair of scissors, and is nervous until they are returned. Yet this is also the child who spends his entire weekly allowance treating his friends to candy and comic books. Or the day before a test he will generously lend out his class notes to a friend, philosophically resigning himself to the prospect of a poorer grade.

Sometimes he is too generous for another's good. Walking home from school, he will regularly carry his brother's or sister's books and coat or will perform the sibling's household chores in addition to his own. He fails to understand that such behavior is not healthy for the sibling, and will insist, "I don't mind. Johnny is tired, why *shouldn't* I do it?" while Johnny magnanimously allows his brother to do his share of the work. In such cases both boys could benefit from a dose of this remedy.

Sulphur at any age can display an astute money sense and sense of value. A four-year-old will accost an adult with the perceptive remark, "That's an expensive coat you're wearing." The boy has a sharp eye for bargains and insists that his parents shop accordingly: "Why do you buy your film at the drugstore when it's much cheaper at the supermarket?" At times this intrinsic sense of value is manifested in more subtle ways. The father of one ten-year-old had been invited to give the graduation address at a state teachers' college. Upon hearing of this honor, the children responded with enthusiasm and praise, all except the youngest boy, who was silent. When the father sought his reaction, the boy laconically replied, "A state teachers' college is all very well, but Harvard would have been better."

Sulphur often exhibits a strong intellectual bent. The boy, especially, has an eager, inquiring mind and from an early age reveals an interest in newspapers, scientific magazines, and, because he likes his reading to be full of statistics, facts, and information, even in such improving works as dictionaries and encyclopedias. An all-time *Sulphur* favorite is the *Guinness Book of World Records*. At times he displays a phenomenal memory for whatever captures his interest. A five- or six-year-old will rattle off the scores and league standings of all the major football or baseball teams, as well as the statistics of the individual players.

Often the boy's talents will run along mechanical lines. He loves to tinker with motors, radios, tape recorders, bicycles for hours at a time, taking them apart and putting them together again, revealing a sound understanding of mechanics. Combining his intellectual and mechanic skills, he also takes to the computer like a duck to water. A child barely out of infancy masters its intricacies seemingly without effort.

In school, at his best, *Sulphur* is the intellectual live wire: witty, alert, curious, eager to ask questions, and willing to answer them even if he does not know the answers; liking to point out exceptions to the rule, or a teacher's mistakes, and to engage in verbal combat. His sprightliness and engaging brightness add much to class discussions. But teachers still wish he would exhibit more diligence and care in his schoolwork. He has plenty of raw talent but, habitually careless, fails to approach the level of performance of which he is so eminently capable. Both at home and in school his innate resistance to authority leads him to devise ways of *avoiding* work, and he will expend more energy on this than it would have taken simply to do the job. Yet when he does choose to interest himself in anything (which is rarely that which is asked or expected of him), he displays surprising application and quickness of execution. Once he gets down to his homework, he finishes it off in an hour, where another would take two. There is a directness and focus to *Sulphur's* approach to any challenge, and his powers of concentration are excellent—albeit short-lived.

At the same time, the rich *Sulphur* constitutional picture

also includes the loafer: the lazy child who cannot be prevailed on to do his homework or even to open a book. At home, too, he shirks his household responsibilities. Even such a small task as washing his own dishes after a meal, taking out the garbage, or making his bed in the morning is a struggle. "Let others do it. I have more important matters to attend to" is his guiding rule in life.

We come now to the *Sulphur* adolescent. Given its heat-emitting characteristics, it is hardly surprising that this would be a prime remedy for teenage boys. Formerly an early riser, the adolescent now wants to sleep in late, then awakens groggy, grumpy, and totally uncommunicative. Although he used to have a good appetite for breakfast, he now wants nothing to eat in the morning, but makes up for it by constant snacking later in the day and eating late into the night. The schoolboy comes home from school ravenous and parched, eager to make himself sandwiches or to snack on cookies and drain glass after glass of an ice-cold drink. *Sulphur* can consume enormous amounts of food and drink; he is the proverbial "bottomless pit." Pizza, in its infinite variety of garnishes and combinations, continues to be a favorite, but the adolescent is essentially omnivorous, liking just about everything, including unusual and exotic dishes. Often he will "jazz up" the food served him with spices and condiments to stimulate his sophisticated (some might call it jaded) palate. Then his table manners (never a strong feature of the type) can be atrocious. Exhibiting an utter disregard for appearances, he eats greedily, even with his fingers, or thoughtlessly helps himself to the lion's share of a common dish, leaving the remains to be divided among several others.

Furthermore, it is often at mealtimes that the adolescent exhibits the *Sulphur* conversational insensitivity. He assertively talks only about what interests him (the difference between his own computer and his friend's more expensive one, or of the problems with his motorcycle carburetor), droning on and on, knowledgeably, but tediously, instructing others in the mechanics of computers or motorcycle carburetors. However, *Sulphur* is also encountered in the opposite extreme—in the adolescent from whom hardly a word can be extracted. He answers questions in monosyllables only, or with grunts of assent or denial, behaving as if every word costs him a dollar. Possibly, he feels a subliminal dread that by talking he might be giving away something for nothing.

The picture of the unwashed, unkempt *Sulphur* adolescent, with pimply skin, visible ear wax, and fingernails bitten to the quick, who constantly pokes at his acne, nose, or skin or scratches his itching scalp is a familiar one. At this stage, too, even his hair may change in texture and become unmanageable: wiry, kinky, growing every which way, as if reflecting the rebellious nature of its owner.

As to his clothes! Believing that his apparel ought to reflect his society-defying convictions, he dresses in a way to challenge decadent "bourgeois" values. If he were to cut his hair or dress neatly, his outer being would not harmonize with his high-minded, anticonventional ideals, and *Sulphur* refuses to lower himself to such gross deception. On the other hand, if he is more materialistically inclined and peer-conscious than rebellious and class-conscious, then he might move to the opposite end of the spectrum. Seeking to outstrip his peers in sartorial elegance, he wears to school the most snappy and expensive clothes in the most current fashion. In one way or another his clothes must make a statement for all the world to see.

The mental-emotional heat of the *Sulphur* adolescent is also familiar to all. More than any other type, he makes his presence felt in the home. Either he is restlessly fighting boredom or he lies slumped on sofas or draped over chairs, right in the center of things. Certainly, growing so fast and changing so much, he might well feel weak and tired, but even this is manifested in a heated form. When a teenage *Sulphur* enters a room, if only to collapse in a chair, the room suddenly becomes too hot and too small.

Then there is his love of disputation. No matter how tired he is, he is never too weak to argue. He will argue about anything—anytime—with anyone. In truth, it seems as if this is his favorite form of communication. "I *like* being argumentative and aggressive," he freely admits, looking forward to the next exciting argument with his family. And if it disrupts the household peace, at least it is better than being bored.

Sometimes *Sulphur* will be critical, uncooperative, dissatisfied even when others are trying to please him. Loudly he proclaims his universal discontent: unfair teachers, unsympathetic parents, too much responsibility, too little recognition. He loafs around the house, seeking quarrels or pulling a disappearing act when most needed. If pressed to do his share of chores, he spends so much time arguing disagreeably that it is far easier for another to do it for him. As to cleaning his room—forget it! "If I were to pick up, I couldn't find anything anymore" is his justification. Adolescents are notoriously untidy, but *Sulphur* is especially so.

Yet the tiresome behavior is more a defect of manner than

of disposition. *Sulphur*'s outlook on life is essentially robust; it is simply that his restless intellectual and physical energies require much stimulation. When they do not find a creative outlet, they can, in the process of seeking out excitement, become disruptive. Furthermore, one senses that the problem is not deep-rooted—merely a temporary stage in the maturation process, which he will (in contrast to, say, a *Thuja* boy) eventually outgrow on his own.

The *Sulphur* picture is somewhat attenuated in the adolescent girl. She is less prone to feeling discontented or misunderstood and, in her person, she is cleaner and neater than the boy. Her room, however, can be equally untidy, looking as if a hurricane has passed through. But the true hallmark of the *Sulphur* girl is the overflowing collection of cosmetics and shampoos—and especially her treatment of the toothpaste in the bathroom. She *always* leaves the cap off, with the paste oozing out all over the sink.

She might, likewise, begin to emit at this stage more heat than before, becoming more argumentative, egocentric, and impatient. As with the boy, her presence in a room can make the atmosphere more oppressive. But on a whole she is easier to deal with than her male counterpart, perhaps because she is usually less purely *Sulphur* and her behavior is modified by some other constitutional picture. It is generally the *Natrum muriaticum* girl who has the more difficult time during adolescence.

❧

On the physical level, a large number of *Sulphur*'s complaints are skin affections. The skin breaks out into hot, red,

itching eruptions of various kinds: pimples, rashes, eczema, pso-
riasis, acne. An unstable circulation, with disturbed areas of heat
(some parts of the body hot, others cold) can be another indication for this remedy, as can certain digestive problems, including a lactose intolerance, complete loss of or excessive appetite,
or weakness or irritability from hunger, especially around 11:00
a.m. Nighttime enuresis or early morning diarrhea are other complaints frequently helped by this remedy.

Sulphur's most prominent modalities are: *worse* from becoming heated, whether from exertion, in bed (the child's soles
burn and he sticks his feet out from under the covers), warm
clothes, hot baths, or warm weather; around 11:00 a.m. - 12:00
p.m.; from standing or sitting still; *better* from cool air; when
perspiring; from energetic talk or activity and intellectual or
manual employment.

Equally important is *Sulphur's* healing powers in constitutional types other than its own. The remedy possesses a unique
capacity to bring latent symptoms to the surface in cases in
which there is a paucity of symptoms to prescribe on; to clear
the system of the effects of previously used allopathic drugs
before beginning constitutional treatment; to promote healing
when other well-selected remedies fail to act; and to prod stagnant cases into progress by reactivating the "similar" remedy.
Finally, the remedy can prevent even non-*Sulphur* complaints
from relapsing or recurring and can help resolve non-*Sulphur*
lingering illnesses by hastening convalescence and cure.

Graphites

(PLUMBAGO OR BLACK LEAD)

In children, the close connection of *Graphites* with *Sulphur* is established by the readiness with which *Sulphur* is prepared to jump *Graphites'* claim in a number of physical complaints—especially in affections of the skin. On the mental plane, too, the similarities are noteworthy, if not as clearly defined. Similar to *Sulphur,* the *Graphites* child can be large-souled and generous-natured (not petty or small-minded), and one encounters the same eagerness to cultivate interests along several different channels—always provided, however, that no single one requires too much commitment. For when it comes to schoolwork, both types are procrastinators and work by fits and starts, interrupting their studies to sharpen half a dozen pencils, engage in some *imperative* stretching exercises, run frequently to the bathroom, and, if at home, make repeated sallies to the refrigerator. In fact, both types can be bone lazy, claiming to be "allergic" to formal education.

But although *Graphites,* like *Sulphur,* is inherently creative, he is not as hardy as the latter type and often lacks its particular gusto. Emotionally he more closely resembles *Calcarea carbonica,* in being sensitive and vulnerable, unable to ignore the pinpricks of life or prevent himself from taking its inevitable injuries too personally. Or the young child becomes beset with a host of (often groundless) apprehensions. If a picnic is planned for the next day, "What if it rains tomorrow? What will we do?" he inquires. If preparing for "Show and Tell," "What if I forget to bring my leaves tomorrow? What if I forget what I want to say about them?" Or, "What if Erica won't invite me to her birthday party?"; or, if invited: "What if she didn't really want to invite me, but her mother told her to? What if she doesn't really like me?"; or, "What if Erica doesn't like my present? What if someone gives her the same game we bought her?" and so on and so forth (compare to *Argentum nitricum).*

Thus the *Graphites* child presents a cross between *Sulphur* and *Calcarea carbonica.* He is independent, but not as overtly defiant as the former; he can be resistant to work but is not as indolent as the latter—and will do at least the minimum without needing to be pressured. And to circumvent the *Sulphur* open rebelliousness as well as protect himself against *Calcarea*-like apprehensions and feelings of insecurity amongst his peers or within the family structure, often the child will employ a tactic distinctly his own. *Graphites* is the family or class clown, who attempts to turn just about any situation into a joke. Clowning around and joking come to him more easily than application; and he resorts to humor to forestall recriminations when he has been shirking his academic or household responsibilities or is otherwise cantering over thin ice. One eight-year-old was a bright enough lad, but an incurable slacker at school and habitually at the bottom of his class. One day he brought home his usual poor report card, announcing with an impudent grin, "Happiness is being *second* from the bottom of your class!" Naturally, his parents could not scold him.

Even the very young *Graphites* learns how to master the technique of playing the clown, thereby diverting just retribution. A mischievous four-year-old girl, to avoid the regulation spanking for running out into the street unattended, would back up into the house, rump first, as if inviting the punishment that her mother now felt too ridiculous to administer.

The *Graphites* sense of humor is not of the jeering, sneering, cutting variety, with intent to demean or ridicule; it consists rather of a well-developed sense of the absurd. To be sure, it can verge on flippancy, impudence, effrontery—and one finds children sailing perilously close to the edge. Occasionally, too, they use humor to stir up others' passions or, like *Sulphur,* to get things moving when life is dull. But for the most part, the *Graphites* humor is more of a shield than a slashing sword, and serves a more personal need. It is the earlier mentioned route of retreat when he needs to extricate himself from a sticky situation. A young child, reprimanded for entering an older sibling's room without knocking first or carelessly dropping a plate when laying the table, instead of getting drawn into a futile quarrel, will draw himself up in mock dignity and composedly throw out, "Well, ex-*cuse me* for living!" And an adolescent girl passionately fond of animals, who would bring sick or dying rodents and birds into the house to care for them, always had some humorous retort ready at hand with which to deflect others' vain protests of "You don't know how to care for them. You don't even know what disease the animal's got."

"That's right," she would reply imperturbably, "and I won't

know until someone catches it."

Certainly, deriving humor from the absurdities of life serves as an aid to self-esteem. One *Graphites* youngster, a budding humorist who had a decided aversion to all outdoor games and sports (in which he alone of all his family and friends lacked proficiency), when asked, "Why, then, are you such a faithful spectator of all the badminton or soccer matches and croquet games?" replied, "I like to watch the players get excited and lose their tempers." The remedy is periodically called for in boys who are physically somewhat clumsy or overweight and roly-poly girls who, realizing they are not going to get through life on looks or outstanding athletics or academics, try to make their mark among their peers by cultivating their innate sense of humor. Without even making a pretense of studying hard or bothering to offer the most basic excuses (and despite being capable of reflecting and feeling deeply), they choose openly to laugh their way through school—and, presumably, later through life.

"There is no cure for birth or death save to enjoy the interval," wrote the philosopher George Santayana; and many a young *Graphites* seems determined to follow this congenial precept.

※

The physical conditions *Graphites* is most frequently prescribed for are a milk intolerance, causing allergy symptoms in the young and acne in the adolescent; stomach pains, relieved by eating, distended abdomen; crusty, scurfy, glutinous or sticky, oozing (also watery) discharges from the ears, nose, and eyes; various affections of the nails: cracked, deformed soft, or ingrown; and, most commonly, skin affections: eczemas, cracks around the external orifices, chapped lips, various eruptions in flexures or folds and angles of the skin (as behind the ears); also, afflictions around the linings of the mucous membranes, such as ingrown eyelashes or blepharitis. The modalities are: *worse* at night; from warmth of bed; from cold; *better* walking in the open air, eating, and wrapping up the affected area.

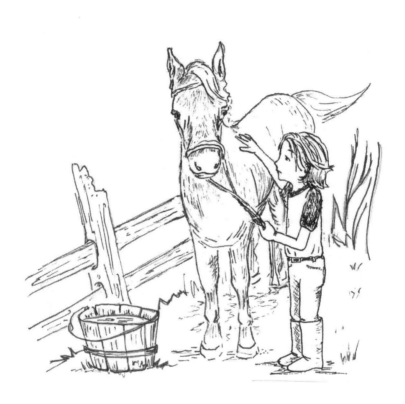

Natrum muriaticum §

(SODIUM CHLORIDE OR TABLE SALT)

T he *Natrum muriaticum* nature is essentially a serious one, burdened by a strong sense of duty as well as a commitment to overseeing the welfare of others. Seldom is the child lighthearted and carefree; rather, he is reserved and gives the impression of sadness—of having come into this world carrying a chip on his shoulder or a deep-seated grievance in his heart. This attitude hinders his exerting the moral influence on this planet that from an early age he aspires to do. For, he must first overcome his personal resentments before he can arrive at that vantage from which effectively to instruct others how to make this world a better place to live.

Natrum muriaticum's archetypal life challenge—that of learning to "let go" of dwelled-on grievances—is the more difficult for him to meet in that, more than any other constitutional type, the child bears the scars of a poor relationship with one or both parents. Because it is near-impossible for the type to express anger in words, he begins early in life to build up resentments which he then nurtures over the years. He suffers from his parents' inability to respond appropriately to his emotional needs, yet he is unable to communicate these needs to them. It is noteworthy and perhaps pertinent that this is the young child who is slow *learning* to talk. With *Calcarea,* we recall, the child is averse to *begin* talking.

Even more: despite his own cravings for affection, not only is the *Natrum muriaticum* child himself seldom demonstrably affectionate, but he actually does not appreciate that which he craves when it presents itself—and at times will actively repel any show of affection. For instance, if the mother takes a job outside the home, *Natrum muriaticum* immediately views this as abandonment. But when she is home, lavishing her affection on her children, he still feels so betrayed that he does not enjoy her presence, as do his siblings.

Thus, *Natrum muriaticum* is not the easiest child to have around. Projecting a "Don't touch me! Leave me alone!" attitude, he later resents it when others take him at his word and do leave him alone. He also pushes away guidance or assistance when most in need of these, shuns sympathy and, when sad, grows angry if consoled—in this way creating for himself a "no win" situation. But to do the type justice, he is acting on some inner compulsion to work through his difficulties alone. This is part of the nature's complexity, not to say perversity. Needing solitude to work out his emotional problems, he rejects that deeply yearned for understanding and affection—and then later suffers from the deprivation.

When the child finds no excuse for injury in the parental relationship, he may seize on some other circumstance early in life at which to take offense. It might be a sibling rivalry or a grade school teacher who is perpetrating some injustice on him; or it might be some friend or relative who does not appreciate

him sufficiently. Other constitutional types in similar circumstances, feeling equally jealous or aggrieved, will fight for attention, argue, or intrigue—or even learn to yield gracefully to the
inevitable. In one way or another they succeed in dealing with
the situation. Not so *Natrum muriaticum.* He might not openly
react at the moment—he does not confront the offender of the
situation directly—but he allows his unexpressed emotions to
fester, and henceforth to color his whole world view. Indeed,
whatever the childhood difficulty, no other type is capable of
extracting a greater feeling of injury from an unfortunate situation, a stronger sense of having been unfairly treated by life.

The remedy picture is prominent in the oldest and most
vulnerable child of the family: the one on whom parents learn
by their mistakes, who has had to hew a path for himself as well
as for his siblings in the family structure, and who thus carries
the heaviest responsibility, whether he seeks it or not. He often
possesses a mature understanding of the relationships among
family members but cannot easily handle stressful family situations. Even if he does not reveal it, he is deeply affected by
quarrels and subliminal hostilities and can become actively ill as
a result. Therefore, although *Natrum muriaticum* could be
viewed as making unreasonable emotional demands, the remedy is also one of the most important ones for legitimate loss,
sorrow, or childhood traumas: neglectful or abusive parents,
severe family discord, an alcoholic parent, loss of a parent through
death or desertion, or parental divorce.

Sometimes the difficult child—or, more precisely, the child
who finds life difficult—responds to hardship by being
ultracooperative, responsible, well-behaved. He is so sensitive
to disapproval and fearful of rejection if he does not please, so

longing for moral approbation that a mere glance from an adult will elicit the desired behavior. When a parent or teacher describes a child as overconscientious, overanxious to avoid giving trouble, or "unnaturally good," there is bound to be some *Natrum muriaticum* in the personality picture.

The type also suffers from oversensitive pride. To admit to error is a humiliation, and to apologize is sheer torture ("I'd rather *die* than say 'I'm sorry'!"). Thus a youngster who has shirked his household chores and been criticized for not setting the breakfast table becomes indignant, angry, and defensive, insisting that it was not his turn. But for the next few days his guilt feelings make him not only set the table without being told but also clear and clean. He admits his error by his actions even though he cannot say it in words.

The child does not cry easily from sorrow. He gets all choked up inside and tears do not flow freely; instead of offering relief, they only give him headaches. He might, however, sob brokenly, in gulps that catch painfully in the throat, from anger, frustration, and especially indignation. In home and at school, during games or in the classroom, he is the one who reacts to small injustices most vigorously. "Hey, no fair! That's no fair! It was *my* turn to be at the head of the line!" he shouts in fury, his face and neck breaking out in bright red blotches from indignation at this miscarriage of justice. Nor is he anxious only for himself. He defends fairness in principle and will rush in to defend others, protesting vehemently, "That was John's ball. Make Tom give it back to John!" even if John is on the other team. Therefore, although the child might appear to be a prig or a tattletale (trying to land another in trouble), in actuality he is seeking reparation for his offended sense of right.

Natrum muriaticum may also harbor an abnormal self-consciousness. Unless he finds himself entirely at ease in a social situation (which he seldom does, outside a limited group of friends), he is all angles and awkwardness. Aware of this weakness in himself, he would like to keep his distance but does not want to offend by being standoffish. Thus, he will be taciturn or loquacious in spurts, first sitting in uncomfortable silence and then, to cover up his ill-ease, suddenly bursting out on a subject that interests him and talking at too great length. Then, just as suddenly, ashamed of his outburst, he relapses into a seemingly moody silence. If he tries to be humorous, it is forced. Or he giggles nervously, laughs too loudly and too much for the occasion, or inappropriately. Even if he does or says the right thing, even when anxious to accommodate or help, it still might not come out quite right.

On occasion, this social unease is reflected in his eyes, which tend to avoid contact with all but the most trusted of friends. Perhaps it is because he fears his eyes plainly reveal his true feelings that he either looks steadfastly down at the ground when speaking or shifts his eyes slightly to the right, left, or above contact level. Just as he unconsciously displays pleasure and enthusiasm by the way his eyes and whole face light up, so he cannot hide displeasure, critical feelings, or disgust. He may not say anything outright, but because his face is always easy to read, the silent disapproval is apparent. This inability to pretend what he does not feel may land the *Natrum muriaticum* child in trouble. If it involves a teacher he doesn't like, his grades may suffer. He then considers this highly unfair, since he has *tried* to disguise his true feelings and has *done* nothing wrong.

At times the clothes betray the type. The child tends to

possess some favorite article of clothing that he wears day in and day out, month after month. Rarely is the girl stylishly dressed. Not possessing the instinct for clothes of a *Phosphorus* or *Arsenicum album,* she is often either overdressed or underdressed for the occasion. Moreover, with so many serious and important matters on her mind, she scorns to indulge in vanity. As with the *Sulphur* boy, the *Natrum muriaticum* girl feels it imperative that her clothes be in tune with her principles and convictions and mirror her true inner self. Accordingly, when in a mood of protest against the deplorable state of this world, her unstylish dress and choice of muted colors reflect this attitude. Conversely, however, the young girl who spends half an hour putting a barrette in her hair or arranging her ponytail in some over-precise way, or in deciding which one of her four almost identical sweatshirts or pairs of jeans to wear to school, is also *Natrum muriaticum.* She will be as fastidious as *Arsenicum album* about some particular aspect of her toilet, which others hardly notice.

There exist strong affinities between *Natrum muriaticum* and the tomboy. Typical here is Peppermint Patty in the *Peanuts* cartoon strip, with her tomboy clothes, manner, and tastes (her passion for and skill at baseball). Also *Natrum muriaticum* is her inability to conform socially or in school despite sporadic efforts to this end, her touching but futile attempts to engage others in serious conversations about friendship, love, and suffering, and who, growing up motherless, is ever searching for closer and more meaningful relationships with her peers.

Although most people like to feel that they are somehow unique, *Natrum muriaticum* children, already sensing their difference and fearing social rejection, seek assurance that their problems and reactions are not different from the norm. Thus, when asked during a homoeopathic consultation about her preferred temperature, season, or time of day, a teenager might reply, "Doesn't everybody prefer the moderate seasons to heat or cold; or the evening when school is over?" Or if asked whether she is habitually thirsty may reply, "Yes, I drink a lot of water, but I'm not diabetic or anything like that, if that's what you mean." Asked about his food cravings, the younger child will reply, "I'm like other boys. I have the normal craving for chocolate and salty chips" (among the type's most prominent cravings). And all the while during the interrogation, he is obviously uncomfortable, sitting tightly hugging himself and looking down at the floor when addressed; and if he happens to be wearing a baseball cap, pulling it low over his eyes to hide his face.

Not surprisingly, in view of his propensity to take life seriously and find life difficult (which is often compounded by an inherent sense of loneliness), the *Natrum muriaticum* child is distinguished by the intensity, persistence, and even utter groundlessness of his hopes and dreams, on which he may live as if they were realities. A city child will spend countless hours dreaming of owning a pony. He knows he cannot keep a pony in an urban environment, but he will concentrate day and night for years on this unrealistic wish, meanwhile missing out on the actual happiness available to him. But then, he may derive more satisfactions from hopes and dreams than from their actual fulfillment. One youngster hoped every year to be elected class president. He finally attained this wish in the seventh grade. Yet the following year he refused reelection, because the distinction proved not so interesting after all (it was just an added burden to his already burdened existence)—and went on to dream happily of someday becoming President of the United States.

Himself, a dutiful child and loyal friend, possessing a sound heart and solid values, *Natrum muriaticum* actively seeks stability and reliability in all his relationships (as against the *Phosphorus* quest for variety or excitement). And yet, despite this trait, his own underlying emotional state can be surprisingly unstable. He oscillates between excessive enthusiasm for and disappointment in people, craving companionship and rejecting it, overassertiveness and a diffident insecurity, a strong desire for acceptance and deliberately off-putting behavior, an abrupt manner (to the point of tactlessness) and evasiveness. Even his affections can be unpredictable. He is subject to ardent, longstanding attachments which overnight turn into indifference. It is as if, having extracted from the relationship all that is needful for his own growth, he is ready to move on to the next stage, and prior attachments merely hold him back.

Just as in human relationships, so with animals. A child will be passionately attached to his pet, for the longest time lavishing on it all the affection he cannot give to humans (in fact, excessive attachment to a pet, especially a horse or dog, is often a sign of *Natrum muriaticum*; cat lovers are more often *Arsenicum*); then suddenly he loses all interest. He undergoes similar radical shifts in artistic tastes. In an attempt to put some chapter of the past behind him, *Natrum muriaticum* will give away his collection of folk music and now will single-mindedly listen only to jazz—or to Bach.

Another facet of the child's unpredictable behavior is encountered in the sudden seemingly unreasonable fits of impatience or the unexpected rages to which he is subject. The normally even-tempered and responsible child, told that his clothes are inappropriate and asked to change them, or who is requested to cooperate with his parents in some small way, suddenly flies into a temper which no amount of reasoning or soothing can assuage. When consoled, the girl might respond vehemently, "Go away! I hate you! I'm ugly; no clothes suit me; and I wish I could die!"

Natrum muriaticum's rages and impetuosity, which seem to come out of the blue, are, however, understandable in the light of the type's earlier described particular pattern of dealing with sorrows, setbacks, anger, and disappointments: not displaying his grievance at the time of the injury or loss—even stoically putting up with a stressful situation—but then suddenly, years later, remembering the grievance (with a passion!) and expressing it on an awkward occasion.

The *Natrum muriaticum* picture figures prominently during the trying adolescent years, especially in girls. These teenagers are difficult not because they are unruly or disobedient but because they are reserved to the point of being introverted and project a profound unhappiness that others cannot assist. Also, the loner streak, which is ever a subliminal aspect of the personality, emerges more strongly at this time. Either because of disapproval of the behavior of her peers, or simply because of a refusal to go along with the crowd, the girl subjects herself to a self-imposed isolation in which she feels both judged and judgmental—inadequate, yet critical. Like *Arsenicum album,* she entertains high expectations of people. But whereas *Arsenicum* becomes angry at those unworthies who do not meet her expectations and, after frankly expressing her feelings, proceeds to disdain them, the disappointed *Natrum muriaticum* cannot confront the offenders. Instead, she bottles up her displeasure and withdraws into herself—and consequently feels even more isolated and wounded.

At this stage, too, the parental conflict might become intensified as a result of the type's strong reforming instincts and insistence that these authority figures mold themselves according to some preconceived ideal. This is bound to create friction. Furthermore, in a continuing reenactment of the unsatisfactory parental relationship, the *Natrum muriaticum* adolescent seeks out authority figures, only to quarrel with them and overturn their authority, once established.

In general, in his concern for the welfare of humanity, *Natrum muriaticum* (an indefatigable "improver" of character and educator of minds, even in youth) is forever trying to influence those around him. Either they are not sufficiently liberated emotionally or they are not sufficiently evolved spiritually; and it is his moral duty to rectify this situation. Thus, an older girl might wish to interest her parents in a New Age self-help group she is attending, which involves shouting out her inhibitions, insisting that they take an active interest in it; whereas such methods of self-improvement might be quite unsuitable to her parents' conservative, old-fashioned tastes. Another type would sense the futility of such persuasion, but *Natrum muriaticum* pushes his reformist zeal to the point where others are bound to resist. Then he feels offended—and grows resentful.

Another quintessentially *Natrum muriaticum* scenario was the college student who, after adamantly resisting parental guidance his whole youth, was now expending much intellectual energy trying to persuade them to follow the teachings of his Indian guru. The potentized salt was prescribed for this trait as well as for the physical symptoms, and he returned six weeks later to tell his homoeopath how wonderfully the remedy had acted and to announce that relations with his parents had never been better: "The remedy completely altered my attitude! I now realize my error in trying to change my parents. I will never succeed, but I am totally serene about it." The doctor was congratulating himself until the patient went on, "During the past weeks it has come to me in my meditations that in my next incarnation I am going to be a guru and my parents will be my disciples. Then they will *have* to follow my teachings."

The young *Natrum muriaticum* evinces many sterling qualities, including a clear perception of and profound feelings for social, environmental, and moral issues, but one of the most difficult life lessons for him to absorb is that just as he insists on being free to learn in his own way and through making his own mistakes, others must be allowed to do the same.

Some pronounced modalities guiding to *Natrum muriaticum* are sadness or grumpiness and slowness in the morning, with a lifting of the spirits in the evening; intolerance of heat and humidity: he is subject to sun headaches or skin swellings and rashes from exposure to the sun, or he feels enervated and depleted from its direct rays. Frequently he suffers from constipation, and in the realm of food, this is the child who likes to eat irregularly and might claim to feel better before breakfast or from skipping meals ("I feel fine as long as I don't have to eat"). Or conversely, the *Natrum muriaticum* headaches are caused by irregular or late meals. His cravings are primarily for salty and crunchy foods (chips, crackers, etc.), chocolate (especially chocolate chip cookies), bread, and soup. He has much thirst, but drinking water or another beverage does not necessarily quench it. Further, with regard to food, the child might choose to make a principled statement which has its roots in some philosophical or ideological belief or in some form of self-denial. Thus, even if he likes meat, he will become a vegetarian out of concern for the welfare of animals.

Other modalities of significance are: *worse* at the seashore; from noise, sometimes even from beautiful music because it evokes longings and sad thoughts; around 10:00 a.m.; from violent emotion, sympathy, or consolation; *better* from open air; cool bathing; rainy days; pressure against the back (and the infant being tightly wrapped); rest and deep breathing.

Sepia

(INKY JUICE OF THE CUTTLEFISH)

T he same cloud that so often hangs over the *Natrum muriaticum* child seems to hover over the *Sepia* one—the same sadness, the same poor social self-image (even while he possesses complete confidence in his intellect), the same dissatisfaction with a parent, teacher, or friend, and feeling undervalued or misunderstood by them, the same feeling that the world is against him or that in some way he has been cheated by life. However, there exists one signal distinction between *Sepia* and *Natrum muriaticum:* the former is frank and straightforward, the latter evasive and indirect. One always knows exactly where one stands with a *Sepia,* as well as where *Sepia* stands on every issue. Also, the type leaves no doubt as to his or her current mood. *Natrum muriaticum,* from self-consciousness, feelings of guilt, unwillingness to injure another, or from trying to "normalize" himself and fit in, often leaves others perplexed as to what motivates him—where he is "coming from" or what he is striving for.

Like *Natrum muriaticum,* the *Sepia* child is usually serious and reserved rather than fun-loving and outgoing, although at times it is a lack of physical energy that makes him reluctant to go out and play. Once he does become active on the playing field, in the gym, or at a party (once the adrenalin is stimulated to flow), not only does he play happily with his peers but he actually becomes bright-eyed and enthusiastic, at times to the point of overexcitation. There is no better tonic for the malcontent *Sepia* than vigorous exercise; and for the older girl, especially, dancing (the type is sensitive to music and frequently exhibits a marked love of rhythm and dance).

Then too, no matter how low his energy, *Sepia* always has enough of it to complain to his family: "So and so is mean to me. Nobody invites me to their house or wants to play with me"; or, "School is boring. The teacher gives us too much homework. And, anyway, she doesn't like me"; or, putting himself down: "I can't do anything right. I'm no good at all. I'm a complete failure," and so forth. This is at home. Outside the home, the child demonstrates a face-saving pride. For instance, when threatened with, "I won't invite you to my birthday party," a five-year-old *Sepia* replied, "That's okay. I couldn't even get to your house. My mother doesn't know where you live."

The child is often clever. The girl displays artistic talent, and both boys and girls not only possess a strong work ethic but actually feel good about themselves and physically invigorated when occupied with mental pursuits. Secure in their intellect, they can grow bossy—the girl playing the governess to her siblings or even parents, the boy attempting to orchestrate family life. Similar to *Natrum muriaticum, Sepia* hates to admit to error (even if a fundamental self-honesty compels him to admit it to himself) and, in apologizing, he feels as if he has somehow degraded his very being. But the same self-honesty compels him to disclaim unearned praise. If complimented by a parent for a picture he drew in school, he will volunteer, "Actually, my teacher helped me a lot."

Sepia can also be intolerant of contradiction, either bursting into angry tears or arguing passionately; and when thwarted by Destiny, he might enjoy playing the martyr. This last is caricatured in the person of the inordinately bossy, but undeniably clever, little Lucy van Pelt in the *Peanuts* cartoon strip, who, when standing by the window with her brother watching the rain splashing against the panes, complains that it *always* rains on Sundays, as if deliberately to ruin her play day. Linus intercedes for the weather: "It doesn't always rain on Sundays. Last week we had a good day...." At which point Lucy turns on him with a black look and a threatening fist, and he quickly amends his tone. "You're right, it *always* rains on Sundays. You're a very unlucky person." And Lucy is mollified.

In real life, this same tendency was displayed in the young girl suffering from a migraine headache eventually relieved by *Sepia*. As her mother was tiptoeing out of the room so as not to disturb her daughter's healing rest, she heard the stern directive, "Don't go running away thinking I'm feeling good!"

But like *Natrum muriaticum, Sepia* is an important remedy for legitimate sorrow, loss, and grievances of a chronic nature— for the child who feels he has been in some way injured or neglected by his parents. (For instance, he might have been left with sitters, relatives, or at a daycare facility while they worked or traveled; or there might be a history of parental divorce.) On the other hand, sometimes the child seems to have brought a negative attitude into this world. Seemingly without grounds he

experiences family life and parental love as a burden, or a gnaw-
ing fear that he is being unappreciated or has been let down by
others undermines his friendships. And it is difficult to get at the
core of his misery and discontent.

Yet the fact that *Sepia* is longing (and is more ready than
Natrum muriaticum) to emerge from the cloud of his discontent can be observed when he receives the remedy. Such a
transformation can take place in this child as brings to mind the
anecdote about the pessimist and the optimist. Two little boys
were sent to clean out a stable full of manure. The pessimist
grudgingly worked for a while, then stopped and complained,
"What's the point of all this? We'll never be able to finish this
job. There's so much left to do, and the work is so boring!" But
the optimist, shoveling away harder than ever, replied, "With all
this manure around, somewhere in this pile there has *got* to be
a pony!"

⁂

The most common physical symptoms of the *Sepia* child are
constipation, lactose intolerance (milk causes constipation or
stuffy noses), headaches, skin eruptions (including ringworm,
eczema, and adolescent acne), a propensity for catching cold at
every change of weather, and nighttime enuresis during early
sleep (so that if caught before 11:00 p.m., usually the youngster
will stay dry until morning). The principal modalities are: *worse*
before a thunderstorm but exhilarated during it (once the pressure breaks); *better* after sleep, even a short nap; from warmth
(but likes cold drinks, like *Phosphorus*); and, above all, from
vigorous exercise.

Phosphorus

(The element)

T he *Phosphorus* child is sensitive, impressionable, finely attuned to another's wavelength. One of his primary concerns in life is to establish and maintain a close, friendly rapport with his fellow human beings. In both seeking and proffering assurances of love and approval, he is demonstratively affectionate, often virtually wrapping himself around the object of his affection, such as his mother, whom he hugs and kisses, pats on the face, or otherwise lovingly caresses, all the while murmuring words of endearment.

Whether actively courting it or inadvertently attracting it, the type from an early age manages to draw attention to himself. He appeals by his alluring looks and bright manner, and especially by his sparkling eyes. Even chance passers-by exclaim, "What a lovely child!" or "Just look at those eyes!" The cry is instinctive, as they gaze in open admiration at a youngster whose alertness, grace, and charm compel notice. *Phosphorus* himself is not unconscious of the impression he is making and can be caught glancing from out of the corner of his eye to observe his impact. From his knowing expression, as well as his ability to ingratiate himself and to please, it is clear that while acting in all sincerity, he cultivates his winning ways.

The light-hearted, ultraimpressionable child seeks above all to be happy. To this end, he does not allow sadness to linger, is ever ready to make up after a quarrel and, if reprimanded, does not bear resentment long. When punished by being sent to his room, he might sing or whistle unconcernedly there, or start drawing pictures. Then he emerges cheerful, picture in hand, and offers it to his disciplinarian as if nothing unpleasant has taken place. He feels the disapproval or disgrace but covers it up, all the sooner to re-enter another's good graces. For in order to be happy, this sensitive child, so highly responsive to others' moods and reactive to their expectations, needs those around him to be so, likewise.

Additionally, no type is more adept at transforming work into play. School for him is a place of fun and excitement where he can daily meet his many friends and endlessly socialize. He even manages to make a game out of homework by illustrating his math or spelling exercises or acting out his history lessons. When ordered to do some tiresome household chore, he does not argue or rebel, but just conveniently disappears. When he cannot evade his responsibilities (a skill in which he often excels), he will approach them creatively. The boy will artistically rearrange the furniture when cleaning his room and the girl will decorate the table she is setting with flowers or array coffee table objects attractively in the room she is vacuuming. In other ways, too, *Phosphorus* refuses to be curtailed in his enjoyment of life. A schoolboy might decline running for office because of the responsibility this would entail. He prefers to remain popu-

lar with his peers and "Free-ee-ee!" to enjoy all kinds of esca-
pades in school, rather than be shackled by duties and possibly
become the target of another's envy or resentment.

As concerns intellectual pursuits, the young *Phosphorus* loves
anything that captures the imagination—the younger child having stories read aloud to him, the older one immersing himself
in fantasy or fiction—but dislikes anything that requires sus-
tained application. For instance, when studying a musical instrument, the gifted youngster will practice eagerly, up to a point.
But then, having acquired the knack of a piece, his concentration lapses and there is little interest in perfecting the work.
Instead, he trusts his innate artistic flair to carry him through a
lesson or recital—which it does! Even though his performance
may be imperfect, he is usually able to charm others into thinking his playing is better than it is.

Phosphorus is seldom mean or bullying. He is not necessarily an angel, but he gains the upper hand in a diverting, not a
disagreeable, way, his mischievousness taking the form of teas-
ing, playing jokes on others, pulling an eel-like disappearing act
if there is work to be done, tricking his elders. A youngster less
than a year old and still unable to walk, will crawl away to hide
in a closet; while others are calling out, searching for him in
concern, he sits there concealed, chortling with delight at his
own cleverness. If an older child answers the telephone and the
caller mistakes him for someone else, he will not pass up this
golden opportunity, but in a most convincing manner will take
on the role inadvertently bestowed on him. A case in point was
the minister who, telephoning one of his parishioners to ask her
to take charge of the church flower arrangements for Easter,
mistook her young son's voice for hers and launched into the

reason for the call.

"I would be glad to help you out," was the ready reply, "but I think that this year, for a change, we should decorate the altar with something different—maybe with some vegetables."

"Vegetables?" was the astonished response.

"Yes, our spring onions are out, and the early radishes, and the asparagus is just coming up—I think they would look beautiful in church."

"But, my dear friend, what *are* you talking about? We can't have radishes and onions as Easter decorations!"

"I don't see why not. Vegetables are also God's creations. And it's time we broke with tradition. People get tired of the same lilies every year."

As a matter of fact, those *Phosphoruses* who do not wear their hearts on their sleeve (and the transparently open child might well be a *Phosphorus)* can dissimulate most convincingly. When the culprit must weasel out of a sticky situation, he confronts his disciplinarian with the most innocent, honest expression, while fabricating a complete untruth. Because of his ready imagination, he is adept at twisting facts or concocting convincing spur-of-the-moment explanations as to why he did not finish some tedious task—and he gets away with the most outrageous lies. With those wide, clear eyes looking straight into yours, you feel he *must* be telling the truth. By no means! The more innocent *Phosphorus* looks, the guiltier he usually is. He has simply practiced his act and raised it to the level of Art. This trait, incidentally, lies in direct contrast with *Natrum muriaticum,* who looks guilty even when he is not, and who always gets caught in the slightest fib. He just does not possess that aura of truthfulness that *Phosphorus* does.

Indeed, when it comes to performing, this type is a natural. Like Snoopy, who, in his antics and serial improvisations, forever threatens to eclipse the rest of the colorful cast of *Peanuts,* *Phosphorus* is the eye-catching, attention-riveting scene stealer, who is ever prepared to dramatize his (or especially her) moods and feelings. The older girl, at the height of elation from being elected class queen or chosen to star in the school musical, might pirouette round the room exclaiming, "Look at me! Look at me! I've landed the lead role in our school play! Oh, I'm so excited, I can't stand it!" The younger girl skips or cartwheels before an admiring audience at home or school, from the excitement of winning a prize, a game, or merely from pure *joie de vivre* ("I'm in love with the world, and the whole world is in love with me!"). One little girl, whenever she was particularly happy, would run outside and dance gracefully around a favorite tree. Conversely, if a *Phosphorus* girl feels ignored, she will sink into the depths of despair. Or she demands attention by working herself up into a state and erupting into impassioned weeping: "Oh, I'm so hopeless and good-for-nothing. I hate the way I am. Oh, I wish I had never been born!" Whatever her mood, she requires an audience to feel fully alive.

Phosphorus children, in general, communicate not solely with words, but with the whole body—with expressive, sparkling eyes, lively facial expressions, mobile features, pretty gestures. And the type's willingness to share with others the exciting things happening in his or her life is always beguiling. Friends and strangers alike respond to the child's captivating manner, and many a dreary life has been cheered by the antics of a lively young *Phosphorus.* L.M. Montgomery's Anne Shirley (in *Anne of Green Gables),* with her flaming red hair and active imagination, and her ability, through dramatization, to endow others' bleak or difficult existence with brightness and color, is indubitably a *Phosphorus*.

Even the younger child can be a seasoned performer. He enjoys fantasizing, play acting, assuming different roles and experimenting with different poses. For instance, he can be impatient, unreasonable, desiring gratification that very moment and, if thwarted, creates a scene. But he is easily appeased and can snap out of his display of temper whenever he pleases, revealing that the act is largely for exhibition. Sometimes he will station himself before a mirror to observe himself crying and raging, genuinely fascinated by his own performance. Even while entertaining others, *Phosphorus* is his own most appreciative audience.

As a rule, *Phosphorus* is prompted by generous impulses. The youngster gives away a toy to a friend or to some "poor child" he has heard of; the older child will spend his weekly allowance on treats for others. What he has, he shares freely— and that which is more rare, will not later resent it (as might the impulsively generous *Natrum muriaticum*). Moreover, he is eager to help out when asked—although, not being the most reliable of constitutional types, he might not carry through. Lost in daydreaming or easily distracted, he forgets all about the commitment he has undertaken. A friend is left waiting for him at some appointed place or a particular responsibility of his devolves on another. Whether this last is true absentmindedness or a convenient lapse of memory is not always easy to determine.

Occasionally the impressionable child becomes unstrung. He laughs too easily, cries too easily, experiences strong extremes of mood, and readily becomes overexcited. He remains

overwrought and sleepless long after a pleasurable event, as
well as from some unpleasantness, and can fall as ill from the
anticipation of Christmas or Hanukkah, a school dramatic pro-
duction, or a birthday party as from the aftermath of these events.
The older child also is easily excited. The girl especially flushes
from eagerness during an interesting conversation or from strong
emotion, and she is profoundly stirred by TV shows, movies, or
a good book, which might cause insomnia.

Phosphorus's emotional lability is one reason this is one of
the finest remedies in adolescence, second only to *Sulphur* in
boys and *Natrum muriaticum* in girls. Physically the remedy
suits both the thin, drooping, narrow-chested youth whose
strength cannot support his fast-growing frame, yet who is restless despite his weariness, and the delicate, somewhat anemic
young girl of lively interests but uncertain strength. Mentally,
the remedy befits the adolescent's roller coaster moods and
emotions, his unfocused, undirected energies—not to speak of
the ardent but short-lived enthusiasms. There is a constant search
for emotional excitement to ward off the boredom that too easily descends on him *(Tuberculinum)*. The girl in particular finds
herself frequently in love or otherwise carried away by romantic
dreams—a state which alternates with despair when she must
descend to mundane reality.

Furthermore, desiring to be all things to all people, the adolescent girl might have difficulty setting the boundaries of her
own personality and needs. In her wish to gratify, and her exer-
tions to make others feel happy and pleased with themselves,
she lies in danger of growing confused as to her own identity.
The adolescent's "Who am I? Why are all these people imposing

themselves on me? Where do *I* end and others begin? What is the *real* me?" are magnified in this overresponsive type.

With his highly intuitive nature and his fluid emotional boundaries, it follows naturally that *Phosphorus* would be the type to evince telepathic abilities: to sense the feelings of a friend or family member correctly, anticipate the contents of an unopened letter, or guess who is calling when the telephone rings. The child might even know exactly what a person, out of sight, is up to, as did the eight-year-old who was brought by her mother for homoeopathic treatment, with her little brother in tow. While the physician was discussing the young patient's recurring sore throats, the boy was occupying himself at the back of the room. Every time he reached out for a book from the bookcase or opened his mother's purse to examine its contents, his sister, without turning her head round, commanded, "Put that book down, Eric! I see what you're doing," or "Don't touch Mother's money! I know *exactly* what you're up to." And once when Eric was about to touch a china vase, the girl cried out, "Don't even *think* of touching that pretty vase!" All this as if it were the most natural thing in the world for her to have eyes in the back of her head. When the girl was not on guard duty, the mother, who had the same ability, barked out restraining orders without turning round. The poor little boy was utterly frustrated. There was no mischief he could even contemplate, without the two *Phosphorus* females of the family jumping in and putting a lid on it.

The older *Phosphorus* child of active imagination might try to read psychic dimensions into every natural phenomenon and aspect of life. A college freshman, who suffered from acute discomfort shortly after every meal, claimed that the dormitory cook must be carrying sorrow and anger in her soul, which was reflected in her cooking. The teenage girl had never addressed, nor even laid eyes on, this allegedly unfortunate person, but she insisted on her interpretation. Once her discomfort improved with homoeopathic *Phosphorus,* she explained that she had meditated daily on the cook's soul and that her intercessory prayers had produced a profound spiritual transformation in the woman, whose food was now permeated with happy vibrations instead of angry ones.

Finally, the nervous, impressionable nature is subject to various fears: of the dark, of being alone, of being abandoned, of thunder and lightning, or simply free-floating anxieties. The child is also sensitive to external impressions. Loud noises startle him, slight sounds keep him awake, bright light enervates; and the changes in temperature or barometric pressure affect his mood as well as his health.

Physically, the *Phosphorus* child's weak areas are the throat and chest. Winter colds that begin with a sore throat descend into and lodge in the chest. Bronchitis, laryngitis, and pneumonia all respond well to this remedy. Additionally, he can be affected by digestive disorders that begin soon after meals, as soon as the food or drink warms up in the stomach; and the most common cravings are for ice cream and cold drinks, foods with a zesty or salty flavor, chocolate, and salads. The most prominent modalities are: *worse* lying on the left or painful side or on the back; wind and thunderstorm, cold, sudden changes in weather; evening, around twilight; also odors, noise, light, and too much excitement; *better* sitting up; being rubbed or massaged; cold food and drinks; and applying cold water to the face.

Finally, in a physical correspondence to the type's overflow of feelings and affections, there is a tendency to excessive bleeding, whether from cuts, from the nose, during menses, or hemorrhaging after surgery (such as a tonsillectomy).

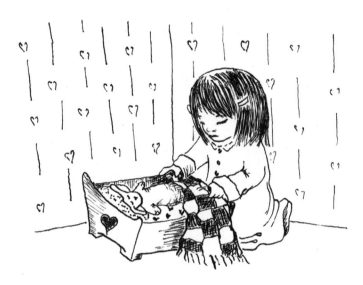

Pulsatilla

(MEADOW ANEMONE)

T he *Pulsatilla* constitutional type is encountered in the child who is mild, yielding, obliging, sensitive of others' feelings—consequently easy to handle. Ever anxious to preserve family warmth and harmony, she (for this is principally a female remedy) assumes a sweet and demonstratively affectionate manner. Climbing into a parent's or an older sibling's lap, the pretty little girl snuggles up comfortably, and remains there passive and content, without wriggling, squirming, or demanding attention—only asking to be closely held. As a result, she is often the petted, pampered family darling, whom others instinctively surround with a protective hedge.

When reprimanded, *Pulsatilla* is extremely anxious to make amends. She lays her head penitently on her mother's shoulder, laces her arms around her neck, and apologizes tearfully, "Please, Mommy, I'm sorry. Please, Mommy, I love you. Don't be angry with me. Please forgive me. I won't do it again. Do you still love me?" No other type apologizes as prettily as *Pulsatilla*, because no type is as completely sincere and devoid of touchy pride.

Moreover, because she relies on others' moods to be happy, no child exhibits stronger peacemaking instincts, be it in the family, at school, or at play. When a cake is divided among a group of youngsters and one slice is smaller, it is often *Pulsatilla* who will accept this portion, saying in the sweetest way, "I'll take that one. I don't mind." Since she generally loves pastries of all kinds, this is a true sacrifice.

Pulsatilla's sweetness and desire to accommodate do not exclude an underlying ability to look after her own interests. Early in life she intuits that if she remains sweet and cooperative, others will hardly be aware of the emotional demands she places on them. However, she is not your typical spoiled child in that she does not grow unreasonably demanding or take the petting and pampering for granted as her rightful due. She is grateful for any support or display of affection and offers love and affection in return.

By nature *Pulsatilla* is shy, with a fear of strangers. In the very young this manifests in an actual clinging to the mother's skirts in public. She hides behind them, peeping out at the world from this safe vantage point. Even in the home she may not venture two steps away. "Mommy, I love you so much I'm going to follow you around all day," pipes mother's little helper in her high, clear little voice, as she trails dutifully behind Mommy through the entire round of daily chores. When she is ill or in need of this remedy, the child virtually glues herself to her mother, refusing to be shaken off. She whimpers if her mother is out of sight or cries when she cannot be held. This trait is reinforced by an innate dependence. Her one great fear is of being left on her own, to fend for herself.

The *Pulsatilla* little boy might appear soft and girlish because of his docile, gentle, clinging manner as well as a tendency to whine too easily. But he eventually outgrows this stage, while retaining a nonaggressive, tractable disposition.

Even after *Pulsatilla* weans herself from the physically clinging stage, she likes to have others take over and relies on their support. Unlike *Sulphur,* she is not one to thrust herself forward in a group to claim recognition ("I did it! I did it! It was *my* idea! Let *me* show you!"), to argue or assert her opinion. In fact, if asked a question well within capacity of answering herself, often she will seek guidance or assurance from a parent or sibling before answering. Nor is she eager to assume leadership. Ever considerate of the interests of the assembled company, she is as content to follow and acquiesce in a group of peers as she is in a family situation. And once she succeeds in overcoming her initial shyness and her trust has been gained, she reveals herself to be a highly sociable, companionable person, relating effortlessly to others.

A prominent feature of the *Pulsatilla* girl is the first appearance of health problems around puberty. Apart from the normal hormonal changes, she begins to develop (perhaps in an unconscious resistance to this first stage of true independence) a host of unexplained little aches and pains: last week in the knee, yesterday in the head, today in the abdomen, tomorrow in the eyes, next week in the back. Nor during this stage is it only the physical symptoms that are ever-changing. *Pulsatilla,* who at any age is subject to changeable moods, now becomes a regular weathercock, cheerful and smiling one moment, sad and weepy the next. The tears well up easily and course gently down her cheeks. But then a word of sympathy or consolation can clear the air almost immediately—the sunshine emerging all the brighter after a shower.

Sometimes the fluctuating moods find a parallel in a fluctuating and indecisive mind. The youngster wants this—No, she wants that—No (changing her mind again), this! In choosing which flavor of ice cream, which doll, which Matchbox car to buy, he or she undergoes agonies of indecision, at length crying out, "Why can't I have *both?*" Or the little girl, anguishing over what dress to wear, turns to her mother, saying, *"You* choose for me." The same irresolution is encountered in the older child who cannot get down to her homework, less from laziness than from a hesitancy about which subject to approach first: math or history? English or French? If commanded, "Begin with math," she starts working obediently, almost gratefully. Even as a young adult, *Pulsatilla* might be unable to decide between two colleges she has been accepted into; which should she choose? She will weigh and agonize, decide and reconsider until the deadline arrives, when she begs her parents to decide for her— and is perfectly content with their choice.

For the most part, then, mistrusting her own judgment and trusting that of others, *Pulsatilla*, whatever her innate abilities, tends to derive confidence from the assurance of others. The dull child needs only to be praised or reassured to become bright and lively; whereas, conversely, the delicate flower wilts under criticism and disapprobation (once again, in direct contrast to *Sulphur* who thrives on criticism and contention). Notwithstanding her insecurity, at times the young girl will display some particular stubborn conviction or a bee in her bonnet. Nothing—no logical arguments, objective proofs, or experience to the contrary—can persuade her that a certain food is not injurious to her health (the child, incidentally, can be a picky eater, suffering from loss of appetite and insisting that she develops stomach pains or nausea from eating), that a certain route is a shortcut to the place she wants to get to, or that some person (usually a male) does not bear her ill will. She gets fixated on some particular idea and refuses to see reason.

One weakness engendered by the combination of dependence and a strong reliance on sympathetic approval is self-pity. This *Pulsatilla* trait can be detected already in infancy in the distinctive tone of the baby's wailing, plaintive cry, which makes one want to console and caress it (not the angry, obnoxious cry of a *Chamomilla*, which irritates). Later, the infant can grow into a crybaby, too prone to wail piteously at the slightest provocation. The smallest scratch must be bandaged, kissed away, and fussed over. Or, if criticized or expected to do something not to her liking, the sensitive young girl indulges in self-pity: "You don't know how much you've hurt my feelings! I can't help it if I feel things more strongly than others." With an aching heart, she may even cry herself to sleep at night, imagining herself seriously ill or dying, with everyone in the family regretting that they did not treat her with more sympathy. Similarly, the older girl is too easily wounded when teased or if even looked at the wrong way. Quick to feel slighted by her peers, she weeps as she recounts her school or social problems. But, characteristically, she always feels better after a cathartic cry. Finally, this is the type that succumbs to elusive ailments as a way of arousing sympathy and receiving the support she craves.

Homoeopathy teaches that frequently a child's outward behavior gives the earliest signs of illness. Since *Pulsatilla* begins early during the course of an ailment to communicate signs of dis-ease in a tendency to cling, weep, whimper, whine, feel sorry for herself, or become overemotional, if these warning signs are recognized at their incipience, much subsequent physical illness can be averted.

ॐ

The physical conditions that most often call for *Pulsatilla* are earaches (affecting either or both ears, especially if switching back and forth); head and chest colds, with bland yellow or yellowish-green nasal discharge or expectoration; loose cough in the mornings, tight in the evenings; stomach complaints, particularly after eating rich or fatty foods or too late at night; loose stool or even running diarrhea; no two stools alike; affections of the eyes, including conjunctivitis, blepharitis, or easy tearing. Also encountered is a sensitivity to heat or stuffy rooms with a desire for cool breezes, an aggravation of symptoms in the evening, and feeling better from gentle (in contrast to *Sepia*'s vigorous) or continued motion.

Other modalities encountered are: *worse* from beginning motion; lying on the left or painless side; getting feet wet, warmth of clothes or bed (despite being chilly); *better* from cold applications; cold food or drinks (though not thirsty); and in the open air. But, it is usually the mental-emotional state that is the primary guide to this remedy, regardless of the physical symptoms or condition.

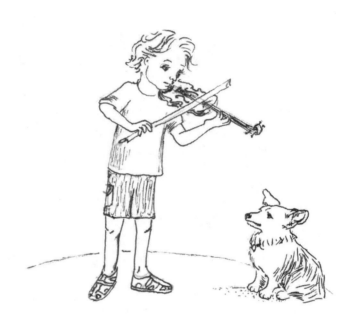

Tuberculinum [§]

The homoeopathic remedy *Tuberculinum* is prepared from the tuberculous matter of a pulmonary abscess, and sometimes the outer appearance and physical modalities alone suggest the tubercular type. The child is of slender build, narrow-chested, with small, regular features and pale, fine-textured skin. He tires easily from exertion, is worse by the damp seaside and better in the dry mountain air, and, despite a basic chilliness, craves cooling breezes and feels suffocated in a warm room. There is a tendency, especially during the cold winter months, for complaints of the respiratory tract to linger, relapse, or recur.

Often a general restlessness characterizes the type. In the infant this can be observed in the way he picks up and throws down one toy after another, tiring of it after a moment—and, in general, never appears to be comfortable or at ease. In the older child, the restlessness can take the form of hyperactivity; ever seeking new stimuli, he resists all forms of confinement. In school he feels like a caged bird, finding it nearly impossible (at times, physically painful) to sit at his desk for long, constantly jumping up on one pretext or another. Bright children find their interest flagging as the school year advances. In fact, lack of perseverance in a capable youngster, a restless desire for change of occupation or environment, and being too easily bored with his surroundings all point to this remedy.

Still older children might begin to complain of after-school headaches and exhaustion. Certainly, there is legitimacy to the weakness and fatigue of the thin, fast-growing adolescent whose strength cannot keep pace with his growth. But then, at the mere mention of going to a movie or meeting friends in a shopping mall, the fatigue vanishes as if by magic and the sufferer springs to life, manifesting boundless energy.

In his eagerness to experience new and varied stimuli, the *Tuberculinum* adolescent, similar to the younger child, finds it difficult to focus his attention for any length of time. In school reading, for instance, he will peruse only excerpts or summaries of the books assigned in class and will resort to (the infamous) *Cliffs Notes* at every opportunity. Even when reading for entertainment he might have difficulty getting through anything longer than a magazine article. Any more substantial text causes his attention to wander and he hastens to seek distraction elsewhere. It is of *Tuberculinum* that one could say that the interests run a mile wide and an inch deep.

And yet, similar to *Phosphorus* (which this type closely resembles), once the child's true interest has been captured, all aversion to mental application vanishes. He is alert, enthusiastic, and throws himself into his current enthusiasm with abandon, experiencing the incidents and events of his life in capital letters. ("You CANNOT imagine the FABULOUS summer job I found. It's REALLY SUPER! My boss is THE GREATEST person to work for and I'm meeting THE MOST FASCINATING people....") Or, often artistic in temperament, he will immerse himself in creative writing, drawing, or playing a musical instrument, displaying undeniable flair. The question is how long will his ardor last.

In his restlessness, the adolescent at times enjoys nothing more than roaming the city in which he lives or the surrounding countryside, even more than hanging out with his friends. Or, prompted in equal measure by a sense of adventure and the desire to escape from the constraints of everyday life, the youth wants to get out and "discover" America or "find himself" by hitchhiking his way through foreign countries. The roving, restless spirit, forever seeking contentment in a place where he is not, travels to satisfy some unfulfilled yearning, some unsatisfied longing or expectation. Robert Louis Stevenson, the writer of children's adventure stories, whose health from youth was undermined by tuberculosis and whose nomadic lifestyle was representative of the type, wrote, "For my part, I travel not to go anywhere, but to go. I travel for travel's sake. The great affair is to move."

In an intriguing physical correspondence to this picture of love for wandering, one encounters the *Tuberculinum* phenomenon of symptoms wandering and ever-changing (*Pulsatilla*). Head pains arise when chest symptoms are relieved; skin eruptions alternate with enuresis; one day symptoms appear in the morning, the next in the evening; skin pallor alternates with red flushes, constipation with diarrhea, hunger with little or a capricious appetite, insomnia with sopor, and so on.

Likewise, the mood can be strongly alternating and capricious. While usually affectionate and agreeable, the *Tuberculinum* youngster, a perfect cherub in appearance, suddenly becomes willful and demanding: begging, squawking, crying, and exhibiting behavioral disorders quite capable of disrupting the entire family dynamic. On occasion, he will even exhibit such destructive impulses as breaking his toys or kicking them to smithereens; or he tries to kick and bite the person disciplining him. In fact, in its role of counteracting in the young child a tendency to outbursts of temper, *Tuberculinum* has no superior except for *Calcarea carbonica* (with the older child, its only serious competitor is *Nux vomica*). The *Calcarea* youngster, however, limits his tantrums to crying, yelling, screaming, and hitting; he does not kick and bite and smash things.

Moreover, *Tuberculinum*'s temper tantrums are distinguished in yet another way: they are accompanied by violent language. The youngster shouts out all the foul and abusive words he can think of. Even a three- or four-year-old, despite his limited vocabulary, will make a heroic effort along these lines, with audacious references to bodily excretions and genitalia.

At times the type's misbehavior is more mischievous than disagreeable. Like *Phosphorus*, the child possesses an impish streak. One three-year-old, having discovered the potential of a really sharp pair of scissors, began to cut out tiny holes in the slipcovers of the living room furniture. Confronted with these misdeeds and reprimanded, he stoutly denied his guilt and put the blame on the family dog, Patches. He realized that as long as he had not been observed he could not be proven guilty, and to make his story more credible, he would, in the presence of other family members, solemnly deliver upbraiding homilies to the mute creature. But there was no malice in him and he admitted to his guilt when it was pointed out to him how much poor Patches must be suffering from being wrongly accused.

As a matter of fact, one of *Tuberculinum*'s pleasing attributes is brightness and a lively sense of fun. A ten-year-old girl would warn her father that smoking, coffee, and alcohol would hasten his aging. One day he parried, "I'm not aging any faster than you, young lady. You, too, are growing older every day."

"Not so," was the ready reply. "Once you're over the hill you start picking up speed." The child had obviously heard or read this phrase somewhere, and with typical *Tuberculinum* quickness she had unearthed it from her memory and produced it at the perfect moment.

At the root of *Tuberculinum*'s restlessness, desire for change, and alternating moods lies the archetypal conflict between the civilized side of man's nature and the wish to be unrestrained. When on his best behavior, the child is exceptionally well-mannered, agreeable, pleasant, thoughtful of others—in a word, civilized. But the other side of him wants to be free to express his emotions and vent his primitive impulses. And this internal conflict accounts in part for the periodic outbursts of temper in *Tuberculinum*'s otherwise sensitive and attractive disposition.

❧

Physically, *Tuberculinum* possesses (naturally!) an affinity for the respiratory tract and is effective in a variety of chest infections that come on during the winter months and then linger (although, paradoxically and as mentioned above, the child likes the cool wind, feels better in the open air, and is significantly worse in a close room); the remedy is also effective in the treatment of enlarged glands and adenoids, swollen tonsils, chronic ear infection, long-standing diarrhea.

But even more significant is this remedy's capacity, in its preventive role, to reach beyond its own constitutional type. If administered to children susceptible to chest conditions *before* the winter cold sets in, and perhaps repeated again in midwinter, it can avert bronchial affections, pleurisies, pneumonias, winter asthmas. It can also help resolve lingering or relapsing respiratory tract infections. Likewise, in severe behavioral disorders that express themselves in tantrums and hyperactivity, *Tuberculinum* can assist types other than its own.

Chamomilla

(GERMAN CHAMOMILE)

A lthough *Chamomilla* does not, strictly speaking, rank as a "constitutional" remedy, in a limited range of common early childhood ailments it does present a personality picture of a highly specific nature. In fact, the remedy could be viewed as the *infant* version of the children's "temper" remedies: the enervated, hysterical *Nux vomica,* the unappeasable *Calcarea carbonica,* or the uncontrolled *Tuberculinum.*

Whether the condition is infant colic (with green stool and diarrhea), teething (with swollen, inflamed, tender gums), an ear infection, swollen glands, or high fever (often with a one-sided facial flush), the disposition is irritable, peevish, impossible to satisfy. He is intolerant of everything. He does not know what he wants—or, rather, he wants many things, but is satisfied with none; then whines, cries, or howls from the vexation of not getting what he wants. And this irritability, which prevents his being at peace with himself, quickly escalates into screaming fits which can, on occasion, bring on convulsions.

The physically restless infant cannot remain still in cradle or crib and wants constantly to be carried. The one thing that brings him any degree of comfort is being carried from room to room, but even here the relief from motion is only temporary. The moment it stops, he flies into another of his tantrums. Moreover, in his unendurable pain (the type is so sensitive to pain that his reactions to it seem out of proportion to his complaint), he might kick and strike out at the person carrying him. His worst time is between 9:00 p.m. and 12:00 a.m. Only after midnight does the exhausted infant finally fall asleep.

In brief, the *Chamomilla* picture is summed up in the well-known homoeopathic dictum that, whereas *Belladonna* presents a picture of turmoil in the brain, *Chamomilla* presents one of turmoil of the temper.

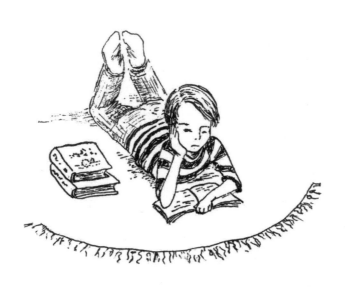

Arsenicum album §

(ARSENIC)

T he *Arsenicum album* child is often pale, frail, and delicate in appearance and, as a rule, high-strung, with a physique that is subject to colds, asthma, allergies and other sensitivities to the environment. But he is not as fragile as he seems. The nature is a strong and commanding one. The child knows exactly what he wants from life and the shortest route to obtain it. True, in his impatience to get where he wishes to be, he might overtax his strength, but even if not possessing as much stamina or endurance as he would like, he can count on an abundance of short-term nervous energy. In fact, although stress and overexertion can bring on headaches, insomnia, facial tics, or digestive upsets, too little pressure can similarly affect him.

A thirteen-year-old *Arsenicum* boy was suffering from fatigue and after- school headaches, growing irritability, and an inability—quite unusual for him—to concentrate on his schoolwork. The cause seemed to be an absence of stimulus in school. He played the clarinet well, but because of his age was in the mediocre junior orchestra instead of the excellent senior orchestra, where he belonged. He liked math and science but for some reason had not been placed in the advanced sections; nor had he been elected to any position of authority or responsibility in his class. Thus, he found himself unchallenged on every front. The following year he was promoted to the fast track in school and to the senior orchestra. This increased stimulus had its effect and all his symptoms vanished.

Ambition is a prominent aspect of the *Arsenicum* nature; the child wants to do well in every sphere of life. From an early age he begins to exhibit a fastidiousness in the way he folds his clothes at night (ever so carefully) and becomes distraught if he spills anything on them or otherwise soils them. He might also become upset if the books in his room are not stacked properly, if his napkin is not folded correctly, if he is eating his cereal with the wrong spoon, or even if someone walks up the stairs in the wrong way—not holding on to the banister as he himself had been instructed to do. There is a "right" way to do things and this must be religiously adhered to.

The slightly older child is remarkable for his conscientiousness in any undertaking as well as for his neat, methodical habits—whether he is painstakingly copying out numbers or letters in his notebook, making certain that they look even; placing the china and silverware "just so" in laying the table, for a beautiful effect; or counting out exactly five grains of food for the goldfish—not one grain more or less. And as he grows still older, he shows considerable self-discipline in practicing a musical instrument and will spend long hours going over and over the same exercises until the precise sound is obtained. He may cry out in frustration or stamp in exasperation at repeated failures, but is ultimately intrigued by the meticulous application this process demands. Indeed, in striving for perfection, the young

Arsenicum will push himself to perform beyond the call of duty.

Finally, the ambitious child can become competitive—determined to be first in his class in *all* subjects. Not satisfied with receiving good grades through moderate effort, he must obtain the *best* grades through superior effort, and applies himself to schoolwork with zeal. For a term paper, he will peruse ten books, where three or four would have sufficed. He prepares elaborately for every classroom exercise or test, studying the material from every angle, or spends days rewriting a three-page short story to make it letter perfect. (This contrasts with the *Sulphur* or *Phosphorus* child, who exerts himself in his schoolwork only sufficiently to "get by.") To such an extent is he driven to be the first and the best in every task he undertakes that the discontented *Arsenicum* is frequently the child who, for whatever reason, has been unable to succeed in some desired achievement and who feels that he is not living up to his potential.

Arsenicum album is frequently endowed with superior intelligence. He is verbally resourceful (selecting his words with care and precision), sharp at repartee; he thinks quickly on his feet and thrives on intellectual challenges. From an early age he can carry on adult conversations with a parent, offering clever, and at times profound, observations on important matters. Not only are his critical faculties well-developed, his mind is orderly, disciplined, and at times refined— functioning like a fine, well-oiled machine.

The child is proud of his intellect. He is a born problem-solver and is resourceful at finding solutions to any difficulty—another's as well as his own. Convinced that he knows best and that his opinions are the most correct (often rightly so), he might grow scornful of ideas not in accord with his own and impatient with or intolerant of incompetence in others. But by the same token, his pride in knowing better than others and in his own superior performance renders him ultrareliable. The child can be counted on competently and conscientiously to care for a younger sibling or even an ailing parent and carry out an assigned task.

Since he must always be right, *Arsenicum album* tends to blame others. If he botches a job, he was given wrong advice; if he performs poorly in music, his teacher taught him badly or the instrument was at fault; if he is mistaken in some piece of information, he was cruelly misled. Further, because he often seeks in life more perfection than can usually be attained or obtained, he can be an incessant and ubiquitous complainer. Such and such is not right for him, that is not good enough; his friends are letting him down; his family, which can *never* do anything right, is composed of "pitiful incompetents," and his teammates, who are entirely responsible for the loss of a game they should have won (had they only listened to his advice), are a bunch of "hopeless invalids." This last characteristic, which the type shares with *Sepia,* lies in direct contrast to *Phosphorus*'s *un*complaining nature. Determined to see the good in and enjoy life, *Phosphorus* tries to ignore the difficult or unpleasant aspects of existence. Demanding of the world's bounty and others' attention he can be, certainly, but he does not allow himself to complain.

Quick and decided in his ways in general, and ultra fastidious in attitude and tastes, the *Arsenicum* child tends also to possess definite opinions, exhibiting an all-or-nothing, black-or-white response. He either strongly likes or strongly dislikes a person, respects or disdains him, with few intermediate gradations. These opinions he voices in strong language. The coach he holds responsible for the loss of some game "deserves to be shot" or his present science teacher is a "complete idiot." Even the younger child shouts angrily, "I don't want to invite Jim to my party. I only want Peter and Matt. I don't care if he's a family friend, he's *stupid*, and I *hate* him!"

To persons fortunate enough to live up to his expectations, *Arsenicum album* is a loyal, helpful, and considerate friend, but he will not waste time on "lowlifes" who fail to meet his high standards. Moreover, with his instinct for making distinctions, he finds himself comparing people for their relative worth. He knows exactly who stands where on the ladder of his preferences as well as in some objective moral or intellectual hierarchy, and does not scruple to express it. Thus a nine-year-old *Arsenicum* girl announced, "Ellen is a much better friend to me than Sophie ever was. She understands true friendship. Sophie was always a loser." Never would a *Pulsatilla* or a *Lycopodium*— both of whom instinctively dislike ranking people in order of merit and tend to avoid comparisons—express themselves in such a way.

Predictably, the same emphatic reactions are exhibited by *Arsenicum album* in his well-defined tastes. He will *love* history in school but *hate* English; like baseball, but not soccer or football. "Football is an idiotic game; soccer is boring. But baseball is different; it has refinement," the adolescent states with dogmatic finality, leaving no room for dissent. Here he differs from *Sulphur* or *Natrum muriaticum* who, even while entertaining strong preferences, always enjoys discussing differences of opinion.

At times the *Arsenicum* child is precociously full of fears and anxieties. He is anxious about punctuality (that he is going to miss the school bus or be late for his private lesson, or that Daddy will miss his commuter train to work); anxious that he will not receive his fair share of whatever is going round; anxious about money. In contrast to the spendthrift *Phosphorus* (and, sometimes, *Sulphur)*, he is careful of the way he spends his allowance (if he spends it at all) and dislikes seeing others spend money recklessly. "Can we afford it?" he inquires of a parent who is contemplating purchasing a perfectly affordable item. "Prudent" is the epithet that comes to mind to describe his attitude toward money, and in the youngster's undue apprehensions one perceives an incipient parsimoniousness. He is also anxious about illness (with an overpowering need to discuss his symptoms) and about death ("Am I going to die?" he inquires fearfully when in the throes of a stomach influenza); or he is anxious about accidents and safety—his own and others'. If he sees a family member swimming in the ocean, he fears a giant wave will knock him down or sweep him away. Regarding a younger sibling venturing some feat, he cautions his mother, "Mommy, don't let Samantha walk on that rail. She might fall off."

It is not only fear and concern, however, that prompt him to issue cautionary directives. Just as often it is a love of supervising and orchestrating others' lives. "Have you got your keys? Your purse? Did you remember to bring along the shopping list? Does the car have enough gas?" a four-year-old reminds his mother every time they leave the house. And at the store he confidently instructs her what grocery items to pick off the shelves. If *Pulsatilla* is mother's little helper, *Arsenicum* is mother's little commanding general, ever ready to take over and take charge.

The type is equally commanding with his peers, ordering them what to do or instructing them how to do whatever they are doing better. And it is usually *Arsenicum* who establishes the boundaries of relationships. For instance, in a friendly telephone conversation, it is he who decides when it is time to hang up. The need to control pervades every aspect of his existence.

Even during the notoriously careless and messy adolescent years, one encounters the same picture of care and meticulousness. *Arsenicum album* cannot tolerate dirt, disorder, or lack of precision. His clothes are clean, his room is tidy, his desk is neatly organized. His very movements are careful and precise and he is punctual on all occasions. Furthermore, in endeavoring to achieve perfection, the adolescent might aim for absolute control over his, or especially her, body. A girl will subject herself to the most stringent food fads or diets and presents the classic picture of anorexia. Spurred on by the type's competitiveness, she drives herself to be thinner than her peers and is secretly proud of how *little* she needs to eat in order to survive.

However, when the *Arsenicum* adolescent directs his or her energies and pride in self-control to worthy causes, one encounters an individual of exceptional abilities, who through talent and a striving for excellence, promises to contribute much to this world.

❧

In the same way that he projects strong mental features, the child exhibits a number of strong physical characteristics. For instance, speaking in general terms, in correspondence to the oft-encountered mental restlessness, one encounters a physical restlessness (with a tendency to pace to and fro or to play with the hands and fingers).

More specifically, *Arsenicum album* is a prominent remedy for asthma, for allergies and hay fever, and for colds with red, runny, itching eyes and a clear, hot, excoriating discharge, which forms a red moustache under the nose. The skin is often dry, itching, burning, flaky, with a tendency to eczema—and there is a burning quality to many complaints. Additionally (and not surprisingly, given its origin), often this remedy is called for in stomach pains, nausea, vomiting, and diarrhea.

The type's modalities are equally pronounced. The child likes mornings. Even during adolescence, when children like to stay up late and sleep in, *Arsenicum* goes to bed reasonably early so that he can leap out of bed in the morning, lively and alert, eager to meet the dawning day. Often symptoms are aggravated around midnight or 2:00 a.m. or the child might experience, regularly, periodic aggravations of a certain ailment (whether daily, weekly, semimonthly, or yearly). Then there is the temperature modality: aggravation from cold air, drinks, bathing, and wet weather, and a craving for warmth in every form: warm rooms, hot baths or showers, warm applications to painful or affected areas, a liking for sunbathing. Some *Arsenicum* children, like *Silica* ones, need to wear socks to bed in order to fall asleep, and if they awaken and cannot get back to sleep, they are helped by a heating pad or a hot drink. Only the head likes cool air, and often the child wants the window open at night to feel the cool on his head, while the rest of him snuggles under a mound of blankets. Many complaints are ameliorated by motion or walking about; or, if in bed, from sitting up or having the head elevated. Eating, also, makes him feel better— although one encounters, likewise in this type, the reverse: the child who refuses to eat, claiming that the food makes him feel nauseous or gives him stomachaches (*Pulsatilla*). Finally, the child is always better from talking about his complaints and from company. Pains, fears, and anxieties are aggravated when he is alone.

Argentum nitricum

(SILVER NITRATE)

rsenicum album by no means has the monopoly on children with a number of fears and anxieties. *Argentum nitricum* is another type that exhibits this particular characteristic.

With *Arsenicum album* the child's apprehensiveness tends to be overt, clearly articulated, and in response to some immediate, concrete situation (his own or another's safety; being left alone in the house for even five minutes while a parent runs an errand; anxiety that he will not achieve peak performance in an upcoming event; and so forth). The *Argentum nitricum* child likewise harbors highly specific anxieties, but the rationale behind them is, at times, more difficult to fathom and the form they take is more covert.

For instance, one child will refuse to be driven to visit his best friend, insisting always that the friend come over to his house. It may take repeated attempts to clarify this seeming caprice before discovering that the child, who has a fear of heights, is terrified that the high bridge they must cross on the way to the friend's house will collapse. Or another child, who has always liked school, suddenly develops stomach pains when he is about to be picked up by the school bus. These will last for an hour or so, after which time they disappear and he can then be driven to school by a parent. Eventually it materializes that the bus is stuffy, noisy, and unbearably overcrowded, and the child feels so stifled and suffocated that he panics. Panic attacks from claustrophobia can arise in a crowded restaurant, a theatre, or an airplane, causing a child to adamantly refuse to go out for Saturday night family dinner and movie, or to throw a fit before the family is about to fly to Florida for spring vacation. The airplane offers no exit in case of claustrophobia and also triggers the type's fear of heights.

Yet another child will one day, without explanation, drop the musical instrument or an athletic activity at which he had become quite skilled and in which he seemed to be happily engaged. Only later does it emerge that this perverse behavior stems from an anticipatory anxiety about the upcoming talent show or field sports day, when he will have to exhibit his particular skill in public.

A significant distinction between the *Arsenicum* and *Argentum* apprehension is that *Arsenicum*'s anxieties do not cripple his performance or impede his achievements. If not entirely overcoming his fears, he somehow manages to coexist with worry and to function well, regardless. The *Argentum nitricum* child's anxieties, on the other hand, can make him less fitted for the world; because of the more hidden motives, his behavior appears gauche, unreasonable, or bordering on the eccentric.

One little girl, whose frequent eye problems had been helped by homoeopathic silver nitrate, had a habit of quietly slipping out of the room a half hour or so after a vivacious, entertaining, popular family guest was visiting, and then disappearing for the rest of the woman's stay. It eventually came to light that the guest's perfume or hair spray was irritating the child's eyes. But the child was hesitant to tell this even to her parents for fear they would bring up the subject and mortally offend the woman, who was something of a prima donna and might well have resented even this indirect criticism of her persona. Another child, also a regular recipient of *Argentum nitricum* for her right-sided nosebleeds, was judged greedy and ill-mannered when, at an extended family gathering, she was observed secreting a box of very special chocolates, brought by one of the guests. Later, when she was chastised by her mother for her uncouth behavior, the girl opened the lid of the box and showed the chocolates covered with tiny white worms. In both cases, anxiety for another's feelings made the girls choose to expose themselves to misunderstanding and criticism rather than embarrass another person. Perhaps it would be more precise to label the *Argentum nitricum* motives not so much "hidden" as "convoluted."

Altruistic anxieties with convoluted motives underlying some form of bizarre behavior are encountered in this type even at a tender age. *Argentum nitricum* was the remedy selected for a bright two-year-old's constant drooling (especially copious in the evening) once his mother related her son's peculiar behavior around Christmastime. At every opportunity he would plunge behind the tree to insert the plug in the socket to light the beautiful twinkling lights on the tree before his mother could get to it. But, because of his drooling and consequently wet hands, he would repeatedly receive an electric shock. Yet, despite cautions, prohibitions, and instruction, he never seemed to learn! An explanation was forthcoming only when one day the mother beat the boy to lighting the tree and he started tugging at her arm. "Don't! Don't you!"

"What is it, darling? Why don't you let *me* light the tree?" she queried.

"Burn! Burn! Let me do it! Let me! You don't hurt!"

In his young mind, the gallant little fellow had linked the lighting of the tree with electric shocks and was trying to protect his mother.

To be sure, *Argentum nitricum*'s deep-seated motives can be manipulative and self-serving as well as self-sacrificing. The selfish or lazy child who wishes to shirk family obligations or to avoid work at home or at school might deliberately start acting in a weird, irrational, anxiety-ridden manner. He has it all figured out: if he acts capricious, incompetent, and irresponsible, less will be expected of him and he will be absolved from his responsibilities. To this end, also, he might become something of a malingerer and claim to obscure head or abdominal symptoms or evanescent joint or eye pains.

The *Argentum nitricum* anxieties are compounded by an overactive imagination—an imagination run wild where impending evils are concerned. The type can be obsessed with a wide range of imaginary "What if?" fears: "What if this oncoming truck swerves and runs me over?" "What if this person approaching turns out to be a criminal and attacks me?" "What if the theater I'm in catches fire and I won't be able to escape in time?" (because of this last "What if," the type will try to find a seat on the aisle or near an exit sign); "What if the tunnel we are driving through suddenly caves in?"; or (as mentioned earlier), "What if the bridge we are crossing suddenly collapses or the car suddenly drives off the edge?" (Compare to the *Graphites* less direful "What if?" apprehensions.)

More disturbing still are the type's apprehensions lest his self-control break down from excessive fear. The older child is terrified to look out from a high window or approach the edge of a cliff lest he feel a sudden impulse to jump from the height. Or, although willing to share in other household chores, he refuses to wash the dishes because, "What if I can't resist the impulse to put my hand in the grinder?" Such thoughts might consume him by day and prevent his falling asleep at night, as he lies in bed contemplating the frightening yet fascinating possibilities.

Because *Argentum nitricum*'s fearful imagination knows no bounds, these children's anxieties can proceed one step further, causing them to become guilt-ridden over some hypothetical catastrophic situation. They obsess over the thought of some past negligence or carelessness on their part that *might* have led to disaster: "What if, that time when I left the window open while I was babysitting my little brother, he had climbed out the window and fallen down three stories? How would I have felt? And how could I have *ever* forgiven myself?" *(Arsenicum album,* who wants to do everything right, can likewise be beset with hypothetical, guilt-inducing worries and fears.)

Finally, one type of *Argentum nitricum* anxiety that deserves elaboration is the anticipatory fears that precede some upcoming event or performance. Despite being well-prepared for a recital, an interview, a test, or an athletic competition, the child is apprehensive of not succeeding and dreads these ordeals. Anxiety robs one youngster, about to appear on stage, of his voice (the throat constricts and no sound emerges but a croak), another of his powers of concentration, a third of his memory, a fourth of his coordination. Occasionally, the child experiences inner tremors or visible trembling before an event. (*Argentum nitricum,* in fact, is one of the principal remedies for these two symptoms.)

Moreover, here again, all these performance anxieties are compounded by the too vivid "What if?" possibilities that rise to haunt him: "What if my memory or concentration lapses? What if I blow it?" These excessive anxieties about messing up a performance or failing in some other way can be so intense with this type as ultimately to bring about that which he most dreads. *Arsenicum album, Silica,* and *Lycopodium,* who also display anticipatory performance anxieties, usually pass through the ordeal well despite their fears.

Another characteristic *Argentum nitricum* shares with *Arsenicum album* is impatience, together with a determination to get where he wishes by the shortest possible route. Both types display focus and energy in pursuit of their objective, but predictably, there are distinctions. *Arsenicum,* even in his impatience, remains deliberate, organized and methodical, confident and competent; there is a flow to whatever he undertakes to accomplish. *Argentum nitricum,* by contrast, is hasty, impulsive, and operates in spurts of intense application. Although focused, he may lack coordination—mental as well as physical; or there is observed a saltation from one intensely pursued project to another.

A child might possess unmistakable artistic talent (usually in the visual arts) and show strong interest or dedication; but the absence of the *Arsenicum* "flow" gives the impression of instability. And if "instability" is too strong a word for *Argentum*'s impulsiveness, it is clear that even if as gifted as *Arsenicum album*—with an equal quickness of perception, nimbleness of mind, and cleverness with words*—the type, working in sporadic bursts, is less at ease with these desirable attributes and achieves his goals less smoothly.

When the child *is* unstable, this characteristic expresses itself in near-hysterical behavior when thwarted or vexed: screaming at the top of his voice in fury, pumping his fists in the air or beating his chest with them; and the younger child might throw himself down and pound his fists on and kick the ground.

Conversely, the stable *Argentum nitricum* child is remarkable for three characteristics: a sharp, observant eye (this is the child who does not miss a trick); a conscious striving to be fair in his judgments; and, in consequence of the first two traits, a fine ability to size up a person or assess a situation accurately.

The physical symptoms most frequently encountered in a child requiring this remedy are: various affections of the eye, including ulceration on the margins of the lid, conjunctivitis; photophobia; laryngitis or sore throats with splinter-like pains; affections of the digestive tract, including sharp abdominal pains,

---

*Thus a six-year-old, listening to his mother and homeopath debate whether a stronger potency of *Argentum nitricum* should be administered for his morning diarrhea before school, suddenly cried out, "Hey, hold it there! Enough of all this talk of potencies. I absolutely *refuse* to be potentized!"

diarrhea from anxiety, strong emotion, or in anticipation of some event, excessive flatulence, and a craving for salt or for sweets, which disagree; overall trembling or tremors in any affected part. The child feels *worse* in warm, stuffy rooms, and at night; *better* from pressure, movement, in the cool open air.

Lachesis

(Venom of the South American bushmaster, or surucucu snake)

The *Lachesis* nature is usually intense and vital, with strong, passionate feelings and an innate intolerance (and, consequently, often defiance) of authority. The type possesses an abundance of animal spirits, which take the form of high physical energy (this is the child who can stay up until all hours of the night and still have full energy the next day), vivaciousness, loquaciousness, or volubility. The volubility, in fact, can be unique; the words spill out faster than the ear can catch, with unfinished sentences tumbling over and interrupting one another, and every expressed thought breeding three new ones, as the speaker jumps from one subject to another.

But the mental symptom most closely identified with this remedy is jealousy. The arrival of a new baby in the family, sibling rivalry for parental affection, or jealousy of one parent usurping the attention of the other can bring on physical ailments in the young *Lachesis* as well as behavioral problems. Indeed, when in the throes of jealousy, even the basically non-*Lachesis* child will often call for this remedy.

The type's possessiveness extends beyond merely family; he resents the siphoning off from himself of any affection or attention he feels is his due. In friendship he, or especially she, demands of others their absolute and exclusive loyalty. That she, herself, is prepared to give absolute and exclusive loyalty in return does not, however, rule out the possibility that at some point she may make a complete about-face. For instance, a girl will adore a classmate, will lavish her with gifts and assist with her homework but then, suddenly, for no apparent reason, might intrigue against her. Then, just as suddenly, she switches back to a fierce loyalty. It is as if the desire is, above all, to keep a relationship at an intense pitch, whatever the means required to do so.

The natural corollary of such behavior is a suspiciousness and fear of betrayal on the part of *Lachesis* herself. Thus, a young girl, trying to be popular and successful in school, might complain of her classmates' competitiveness, envy of her accomplishments, intrigues, disloyalties, and lack of trustworthiness. This clearly mirrors her own feelings and behavior which, in self-justification, she attributes to her friends. The type's distrust is often reflected in the eyes. Not only does the child possess a quick, alert, knowing glance, but also a darting, sidelong, mistrustful one. Or he peers suspiciously out from under half closed lids or from the corner of his eye.

But the serpent mentality is nothing if not labyrinthine, so that alongside of this suspiciousness of people, the young *Lachesis* also possesses a keen awareness of their true nature. He displays a capacity to go straight to the heart of another's strength or weakness, penetrate his motives, and anticipate his actions and reactions. In this way he is able not only fully to empathize with another but, even more significant, he is able to forge those intense friendships that are so meaningful and important to him— and which can, despite occasional setbacks, last for years.

One likewise encounters in the *Lachesis* child a manner that appears to be quite the reverse of the intense, loquacious, strongly projecting personality: a shyness and reserve. In actuality these traits mask a passionate nature and an inquiring mind—an eagerness to master life's complexities and understand its paradoxes by quietly observing (like the coiled, still-lying, but ever-watchful snake). And that which betrays the type is the above-mentioned sharp, observant eye; also the way in which once launched on a topic of particular interest (frequently one that comprises some moral conflict), even the habitually laconic *Lachesis* youngster will express himself in a rush of unarrestable words, at times exhibiting an extraordinary command of language.

Such was the quiet eleven-year-old girl, subject to severe after-school headaches. She had long been preoccupied with the moral issues raised in the study of history, and at present she was especially intrigued by the Middle Ages, which she was studying in class, and by the paradoxes of Christianity. Was the church militant, a progressive or regressive influence on European civilization? Did it spread culture and learning and civilized behavior or did it breed ignorance, superstition, and war? And was this paradoxical influence true of other great religions of the world? These truly difficult concepts the child sensed and was trying to understand. (No wonder she had those after-school headaches!)

Only the mature mind can appreciate relativism and paradoxes and sense moral conflict. And it is of *Lachesis* children that it can be said that they are wise beyond their years or "born old," because, from an early age, they appear to possess something of the wisdom of the serpent. This, in fact, could be one of the reasons the "constitutional" type is encountered in young children only occasionally—and then, more frequently in girls who, as a rule, mature more rapidly than boys.

Beginning already with the toddler, *Lachesis* girls can be remarkably bold, articulate, and imperious. They will fearlessly walk up to strangers and engage them in adult-like conversations; they do not hesitate to express not only their wants but also exactly how they feel about these wants and the reasons they should be heeded; and they boldly and frankly state their opinion of others' behavior.

A four-year-old, usually of a peaceable disposition, had suddenly undergone an inexplicable transformation and was striking out at her siblings verbally and physically, like a veritable snake. When sternly reprimanded, then punished for her unacceptable behavior, she lashed out at her parents with verbal venom. "You are animals—nothing but wild animals! You are worse than animals. Animals at least love their young and don't punish them like you do. You are not only animals but *real beasts!*" (Note her precocious feel for the distinction between the two words.) She was beside herself and carried on like this for days. At one point, when her unruliness provoked the threat that Santa Claus would not remember her at Christmas, she responded with the defiant declaration, "I don't care! I *hate* Daddy, Mommy, God, *and* Santa Claus!" Yet, the internal struggle was quite visible: "I want to be good. Part of me wants to be good and tries hard, but something in me *makes* me bad. I hate the bad part, but I can't help it...." she would sob, as if some inner force was driving her to disruptive behavior.

A dose of *Lachesis* was administered and she was sent up to her room. An hour later she came down and announced quietly and simply that she was over her "badness" and would be "good—forever." And she lived up to her word. Purged of whatever destructive force was possessing her, the tantrums never returned and, henceforth, she took on the role of peacemaker in the family—a striking example of *Lachesis's* defiant, disruptive energies being transformed into cooperative and creative ones.

Frequently a trenchant sense of humor characterizes the type. If *Graphites* is the class clown, *Lachesis* is the class wit, whose clever quipping and stinging remarks secure for him a powerful position in the class. Yet just as often, the child uses his rapier-like wit to depersonalize his hardships or mask a barely tolerable family situation.

The case of an adolescent boy rebelling against school and studies offers a perfect example of several *Lachesis* traits, including this last. He was brought, protesting, to a homoeopath, ostensibly for a tendency to painful throat infections (he described the characteristic *Lachesis* sensation of a lump in the throat with the words, "Swallowing is like passing over a mountain"), but in reality for a tendency toward disruptive and defiant behavior in school. Although obviously intelligent, he was failing in his courses and totally lacked any sense of responsibility with regard to his studies, handing in his homework late (if at all) and shirking all classwork. Instead, he spent his time in class cracking jokes, making humorously deprecating remarks about school, and ridiculing the teachers. True, the family situation was not an easy one: his parents were undergoing an ugly, protracted divorce, and one sibling was disabled. But although this could explain, it did not justify his wasting his own and others' time in class, and, with his cutting tongue and rabble-rousing proclivities, he was inciting his classmates to a similar rebelliousness.

He also possessed the type's suspicious yet intuitive nature. Suspecting that it was not only for his sore throats that he was undergoing homoeopathic treatment, and intuiting the remedy about to be administered, he threw a sidelong glance at the physician, protesting, "I don't want you to give me snake poison or anything like that." And after receiving the medicine under his tongue, he promptly tried to spit out the (fortunately) rapidly dissolving granules.

For several ensuing weeks there was no sign that his papers would be handed in on time, nor that his attitude would change. But then one morning he awoke and, setting aside rebellious proclivities, resolved to apply himself to his books. "I don't know why I made that decision," he later said. "It was like suddenly deciding to give up smoking." This was his only explanation of the subtle action of *Lachesis* on his psyche.

ঞ্চ

In children, the physical conditions that most frequently call for this remedy are throat inflammations or infections (primarily left-sided, with a feeling of a lump in the throat, making empty swallowing painful or difficult, but better swallowing solids), sometimes with a sharp, stabbing pain in the ear; left-sided frontal or eye headaches that are throbbing, pounding, or coming on in waves of pain; excessive bleeding from the nose or from cuts (when *Phosphorus* is unavailing), and serious skin and septic infections, with purple, dark red, bluish-blackish discoloration to the ulcers, boils, swellings, etc. In any of these acute conditions, no collaborating mental-emotional symptoms of *Lachesis* are required.

The principal modalities encountered in children are: *worse* after sleep (the child wakens into an aggravation), in the morning; from the heat of summer, the sun, stuffy rooms, hot drinks (this is the child who, like *Sulphur,* generates physical as well as emotional heat); from pressure of clothes (particularly round the neck and waist); *better* at night, from laughing, crying, talking (the child can "talk away" almost any difficulty or problem); from cool bathing (especially of the affected part), the open air, cold drinks. Finally, the child's night energy is a marked feature.

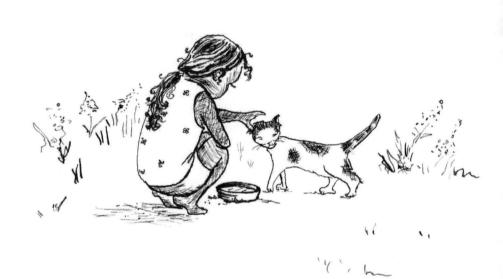

Medorrhinum

T he *Medorrhinum* nature is a complex one. On the one hand, exuberance, enthusiasm, forcefulness, and high energy mark the type—traits that nourish productivity and talent. On the other hand, when the same energy is misdirected, the child can be manipulative, selfish, and unruly.

In the early years, the child is constantly touching things, knocking them over, tripping over himself in his haste to gain his immediate desire—at times with an utter disregard for safety. This heedless behavior is actually a reflection of a deeper stratum of the personality—of the way in which *Medorrhinum* absorbs knowledge and information. The type must *act out* the information before it is creditable or even comprehensible, because with him, knowledge is born of action and must be experienced in action. Even the bright *Medorrhinum* youngster cannot learn from being told that the stove is hot, but must burn himself (more than once) before anticipating the consequences of touching it. Throwing caution to the wind, he acts rashly, reacts immoderately, speaks up boldly, or pushes events and situations to the breaking point to learn what he can or cannot do.

The older child is impatient as well as impulsive. He invariably attempts to hasten events to their resolution, getting angry at delays and frustrated when a project is not accomplished by yesterday. This characteristic does not, however, prevent his being a procrastinator. A methodical approach tires his patience, and he tends to postpone things until the last moment, at which point he is forced to operate under pressure. Typically, a schoolboy will put off all the weekend (and, when he can manage it, the week's) homework until Sunday evening. Then he works in haste, late into the night. Yet somehow he succeeds in completing the assignment on time *and* receiving decent grades. He accomplishes this because, unmethodical work habits notwithstanding, on a certain level some mental process has been gradually unfolding. The *Medorrhinum* pattern is to harbor a vague inspiration, put it aside, recapture it, put it aside again, and let it simmer in the back of his mind. Then all of a sudden, under pressure, the ideas, welling up after long simmering, come together in a coherent end product. In fact, when the energy-generating pressure is missing, the child finds it difficult to concentrate and his performance is flat.

The hurried, spasmodic cast of his mental output is often exhibited in a child's speech. He expresses himself in hasty spurts, as if fearing to lose his train of thought or rush of inspiration. With his impulsive thoughts springing seemingly from nowhere and ending everywhere, *Medorrhinum* is one of the constitutional types that, like *Sulphur,* loves *talking* the world to rights. If this requires many words, so much the better. Occasionally, his speech reflects a mental confusion. The child repeats himself or leaves sentennces unfinished, or, like *Thuja*, forgets words or ideas.

At times the release of intense energy expresses itself in disruptive behavior. The child is a troublemaker: not as overtly disruptive as *Tuberculinum,* but more scheming and under-handed—always causing confusion, which he then revels in. In his own eyes, of course, this behavior is justified, since he labels as "hostile" anyone who protests his behavior, interferes with his desires, or does not accede to his demands. All means are permissible in self-defense.

The young *Medorrhinum* who is manipulative, egotistical, and difficult to manage often becomes so from a loss as to where to direct his energy constructively. When this type does turn his attention to a worthy cause, he does so in a conscientious and unsparing manner. Aggressive behavior was encountered in an eleven-year-old boy, small for his age, which circumstance had a deleterious effect on his disposition. To offset his half-pint size he became the neighborhood bully, picking on any child younger or weaker than he. *Medorrhinum* prescribed several times over the course of two years did not affect his growth much, but his disposition altered markedly for the better. He now became the protector of younger children instead of their oppressor, and guarded over them to ensure that no one else bullied them.

Medorrhinum can be exceptionally sensitive and compassionate toward those of his fellow creatures (both human and animal) on whom he has chosen to lavish his attention. An endearing example was the twelve-year-old girl who, although a disruptive influence in the home, expert at pitting one family member against another, was exceedingly considerate of animals and felt it her obligation to see to the welfare of the neighborhood dogs and cats. Winter and summer she would conscientiously set out pans of water for them and dutifully refill them twice a day. She would also offer to walk any dog whose masters worked all day. This tending to others' pets was no passing whim, but a charitable impulse that continued for years, eventually culminating in a degree from veterinary school.

Unlike the focused *Arsenicum album* and *Nux vomica,* who always know exactly what they want, *Medorrhinum* is often unfocused, aware only that an inner force is driving him to some unclear end. This uncertainty might render him impatient, disruptive, selfish. For this child needs to be clearly challenged. Then, to meet a particular challenge, he will respond with energy, enterprise, and dedication.

ঽ৲

The physical conditions that are most often encountered in the type are chronic or recurring upper respiratory tract ailments (stuffy noses and congested sinuses, with a thick, tenacious, green mucous discharge); a fishy or briny odor to the excretions; nighttime enuresis; joint or bone pains (when other remedies fail to act). *Medorrhinum* is also prescribed for infant asthma and for children stunted in growth but of strong ego. Pains are usually *worse* in a close room (like *Pulsatilla* and *Tuberculinum),* before thunderstorms (like *Sepia),* and from sunrise to sunset. They are *better* from sunset to sunrise and at the seaside; also from fresh air, from stretching, from strong pressure, or when lying on the abdomen.

The remedy is prepared from the gonorrheal bacteria.

Lycopodium

(CLUB MOSS)

Because there is frequently a mature quality to the *Lycopodium* personality, in children the constitutional picture (in contrast to the acute or primarily physical one) tends to emerge with age, usually more often in boys than in girls.

An inherent self-esteem characterizes the type. Intellectual pursuits come easily to the boy; sometimes it seems as if he imbibes knowledge purely by osmosis. He is capable of talking intelligently about history he has never learned or books he has never read, but which he has heard discussed by his elders. Consequently, he feels himself to be strong, capable, and worthy of respect. A self-respecting ten-year-old who was good at drawing was the son of a rather prominent government official. One day his father jokingly encouraged him, "Keep up your drawing, Henry, and someday you will be well-known as the gifted son of the famous Joseph N___."

"No, Dad, you've got it backwards" was the cool reply. *"You will soon be known as the gifted father of the famous artist,*

Henry N___." The seriousness and self-assurance behind the humor were evident.

The good image *Lycopodium* entertains of himself—his supreme (although not always justified) self-confidence—compels others to think well of him also. And it is further strengthened by a grounded, balanced attitude toward life, where he does not expect too much from his fellow human beings or make too heavy emotional demands on them. Further, although self-willed, the child senses the futility of discord or rupture and is usually adept enough to judge exactly how far he can push. Unlike *Sulphur, Medorrhinum,* or *Nux vomica,* who in their self-assertiveness often appear to be "cruising for a bruising," *Lycopodium,* even when eager to assert his will, knows when to yield—when not to pit himself against stronger forces. This trait was exhibited in a boy whose sixth-grade English teacher, believing his grade book to have been stolen by one of the pupils, announced to the class that unless it was returned, he would have to decide arbitrarily what grades to give out. The book was not returned and the boy got a C+ on his report card. Surprised, he took his compositions and tests to the teacher to show that he had gotten all A's and B's; but the latter, for reasons of his own, stuck by the grade.

After an initial justifiable anger and frustration, which according to his parents lasted only a few minutes, the boy shrugged his shoulders and said, "Oh, well, what the heck!" and there the matter ended. He later explained, *"I* know that I got all A's and B's and did well in the course, so what do I care if the teacher gave me a C+? I suppose it's his way of getting back at me. I certainly was no angel in class this year." He was self-respecting enough not to remain vexed at another's unfair or irrational conduct. Such a mature reaction lies in direct contrast to the fury and indignation a *Natrum muriaticum* would evince at such treatment; and who months or even years later would recall with passion the injustice perpetrated on him.

Lycopodium is also adept at deflecting recriminations. When caught in some misdemeanor, he will say, "Sorry! Sorry!—I said, 'I'm sorry.' What else do you want me to say?" in a tone implying that the other is being petty or unreasonable to be upset by or even notice such a trifle. Or, when corrected in a flagrant mistake of judgment or opinion, he immediately cuts short the person rebuking him with a cavalier "Okay, okay, so I was wrong *this* time. So what? Everyone has a right to be wrong once in a while!" —and proceeds to change the subject.

The *Lycopodium* girl can be equally unflappable. Finding herself in the wrong, she will apologize without conviction, proffer some perfectly logical and self-exonerating reason for being so, or offer a sensible suggestion how to remedy the error— then tranquilly go on with her life. A seven-year-old girl, about to be rebuked for being too imperious with her brothers, addressed her mother with perfect composure, "Mommy, before you get excited about this issue and drag in the whole family, let us first talk about it calmly, woman-to-woman." Preserving emotional detachment ("keeping cool") is extremely important to a *Lycopodium,* and all his instincts go out to cultivate this trait.

To this end he will, for example, avoid making distinctions between people. He treats them all evenly and equally, restraining himself from showing favoritism. This contrasts with *Arsenicum album,* who is always comparing and contrasting people, thereby displaying his attachments, and with *Natrum muriaticum,* who can never cultivate dispassion in his relationships. Furthermore, it is in order to remain detached from strong emotion that *Lycopodium* will exercise his often pleasing wit. For instance, a boy out on a family expedition to buy plants for their flower boxes (when every member is vying loudly for his or her choice of pansy or petunia) will disperse the growing acrimony by suddenly backing off at the height of the heated discussion and wearily remark, "I forgot how much fun it is to go shopping with the family!"

Even the toddler senses the power of wit to deflect emotional heat. A youngster not yet three, hearing his two elder sisters arguing over a pink cardigan ("It's mine!" "No, it's mine!"), quickly joined the fray and, stamping his foot, cried out in mock anger, "No, it's mine!" Both girls instantly turned on him in indignation at this disrespectful interruption of their dispute, but then burst into laughter.

All this contributes to *Lycopodium*'s aura of being good-natured and easy to deal with. Provided he is not seriously crossed, he is often just that. But being highly conscious of power, his cooperativeness and accommodating manner stem more from the head than, like *Pulsatilla*'s, from the heart. In fact, it is during these early years, when he is learning how to jockey for positions of strength, that the groundwork is laid for the arrogance that emerges with age, and for which the type is renowned.

He is arrogant in the way *Sulphur,* for example, is not. *Sulphur* can be the boastful, aggressive entrepreneur who insists on going his own way, but others are free—are even generously invited and encouraged—to join him in his enterprises and share in his glory. The same cannot be said of the *Lycopodium* who has reached a position of eminence. Once there, he brooks no competition or companionship. Even though willing to be of assistance, in his leadership capacity and sense of supe-riority he remains somewhat aloof.

To claim that all *Lycopodium* children fit this sanguine, self-esteeming picture would, however, be an oversimplification. There does exist a more fearful or cautious type, closer to the insecure *Calcarea carbonica* picture than to the rugged *Sul-phur* one. Glancing warily out from under a furrowed brow, this is the child who carefully sizes up a situation or a person before acting or responding and, being highly conscious of the impression he produces on others, is judging how not to make any misstep. Sometimes he so cautiously weighs his words be-fore he commits himself to anything that he gives the impres-sion of being self-serving—which he can be; just as he can be unruly, ill-humored (the young child wakes up cross and quar-relsome in the morning), dictatorial (the older child insists on ruling the roost and allows for no other ways but his own), and, above all, headstrong (not to be deflected from his chosen course of action). But even his dissatisfaction or displeasure is more often reserved than explicit, exhibited more by a pained ex-pression or a frown or a contemptuous tone of voice than in a tendency to whine or complain. And as a rule, he is slow to anger; although, once ignited (primarily when opposed), he can go off like a Roman candle and is blind to reason, unreachable by any persuasion. For the most part, however, *Lycopodium* will project an image of self-possession, self-containment, self-respect—a picture that befits a future leader of men.

❧

The physical symptoms in infancy and childhood for which *Lycopodium* can be prescribed even without the confirmatory mental picture are: colicky stomach pains; strong sweet cravings or hunger at night; a capricious appetite—either the child feels filled after a few mouthfuls but then hungry an hour later, or the appetite increases the more he eats, and he does not know when to stop; excessive flatulence; eczema; chest colds with tenacious coughs; and especially right-sided tonsilitis and sore throats—all with the typical 4 to 8 p.m. aggravation of symptoms.

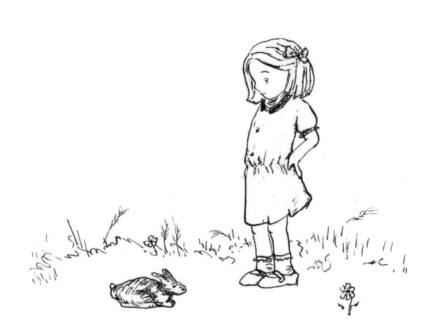

Causticum

(HAHNEMANN'S SPECIAL PREPARATION OF LIME AND BISULPHATE OF POTASH)

S imilar to *Lycopodium,* the *Causticum* child gives the impression of being well-balanced, both socially and emotionally, with his manners and temper under good control. Like *Lycopodium,* too, he feels at ease in most social situations, and (most significant), innately accepting human nature as is, he possesses a talent for making others feel comfortable in his presence. He also knows how to cooperate in a group; is himself energized, not depleted, by peer companionship; and in fact, regards a day without socializing as a day not worth living.

Causticum's social adroitness stems from not only a fine attunement to another's sensibilities but also a sympathetic nature—a characteristic he possesses in abundance, at times to the point of becoming too easily upset over others' pains or problems. For example, the child might develop physical symptoms (something as concrete as joint pains) following a quarrel between family members or between friends, even if it does not concern him directly. Or he gets too deeply or lastingly involved in children's sandbox wars. This sympathy can extend to all living creatures. A woman was relating how her eight-year-old daughter was, alone in the family, strictly vegetarian. "We as a family are more or less vegetarians. That is, we like to consider ourselves 'polite vegetarians,' eating what is served when dining out. Deborah, however, will not compromise. In fact, as soon as she learned to speak she would, when eating meat, inquire, 'What's it made of?' When told that the meat came from a chicken or a lamb, she would start crying and say, 'Poor chickie!' or 'Poor little lamb!' and push away her food, untasted."

And another slightly younger *Causticum* girl would become upset when some insect or bug was swept out of the house or even wiped off her person, for fear it might be injured ("Don't brush it off, Mommy. Let it stay. I don't mind—really. Brushing it off might hurt it."). Once, at a family picnic, she even protested the brushing away of a colony of ants advancing towards the leftover food, crying out, "Don't do that! They must be hungry! Don't they have as much right to the food as we do?"

Like *Natrum muriaticum,* the *Causticum* child might begin early in life to sense the essential sadness in this world and exhibit periods of melancholy. The difference is that *Natrum muriaticum's* sadness is more deep-seated and tenacious, and affects the whole of his outlook on life; whereas with the more balanced *Causticum,* sadness has its place in the overall scheme of things. Even if felt acutely at the moment, or lingering for some time, sadness does not cause a distortion that will permanently affect his world view. When circumstances change, his attitude rights itself and a more cheerful outlook prevails.

The type is not without its own particular weaknesses, however, the principal one of which is, with age and a growing security of social standing (and without entertaining overly high expectations of others' capacities), the child may become opinionated. This is not the *Arsenicum album* or *Nux vomica* who knows better than another about a given subject; nor is it the *Sulphur* boastfulness about some specific accomplishment. *Causticum* confidently airs his (not necessarily informed) opinions about *everything* and is ready to give advice to anyone— even to the expert in his own field. Thus an adolescent who knows very little about music will say to a friend who plays in the school band, "I don't see why on earth you bother with the saxophone, even if you do enjoy it. There is a much greater demand for the guitar. Also, you've got a good voice and then you can accompany your own singing if you want to earn some money..." Or another adolescent will challenge an older sibling who has decided which college to attend: "Why did you choose x? With your interest in architecture, you should really have chosen y or z, both of which have better art departments. Although I, personally, think you'd do better in engineering. Take it from me, that's where your real talent lies."

If *Causticum* is quarrelsome, it is not from selfishness, an unreasonable willfulness, or anger at being thwarted in his designs, it is precisely because his opinions are being challenged. (*Lycopodium* has every bit as high an estimate of his own opinions and does not easily tolerate contradiction, but he is not as obvious about it; instead of quarreling, he hides his displeasure under an air of superior indifference or disdain.) But although this type might appear too insistent in his views and his ideas on management of his life, from being inherently sensible and conscientious (an old head on young shoulders) he tends to judge correctly what is best for him. Authority figures may well

leave him to make his own decisions as early as age permits—
and allow him to pursue his own course, even if this entails
making a few mistakes. (Let him learn that he is not *always*
right.)

One additional difference between this child and *Lycopodium* should be noted. *Causticum* is "strong on justice." He
expects the world and people to be just and, contrary to the
above mentioned acceptance of people, grows dismayed when
justice does not prevail. *Lycopodium* either instinctively senses
the inevitable injustices of this world or simply is less concerned
about justice. With him, the important point is not to permit
himself to become distraught over this particular realization—
but, accepting it, try to work with and through it to a higher
good. This is how, later in life, he succeeds in the world of
politics, law, and large institutions. Conversely, *Causticum* (like
Natrum muriaticum) makes his mark in the world by actively
pitting himself against injustice.

Concluding with the mental-emotional picture of *Causticum*,
one point to be borne in mind is that the child's impulses generally are benign. Even his tendency to be opinionated stems
from a desire to assist erring humans resolve their problems or
an off-balance world regain its equilibrium. This fundamental
goodwill, combined with friendliness, an essentially balanced
disposition, and a well thought through approach to life (he is
one cautiously to test the waters before committing himself),
causes the remedy to be prescribed to children primarily for
some specific physical complaint rather than a behavioral disorder or emotional imbalance.

A boy of four was brought to a homoeopath for twitchings
and jerkings at night in bed. The overall physical picture sug-

gested *Causticum,* and the physician, casting about for confirmatory mental symptoms, inquired of the mother whether her son had any particular stress in his home or nursery school to cause the nervous twitchings. At first she could not identify any stress, since the boy—the youngest of four children, adored by parents and siblings alike—was still at a stage in life wherein he felt as assured of happiness and never-ending love around him as of the supply of air and sunshine.

"No stress that I am aware of," she replied, her mind drawing a blank. "Life to Jamie is one long carnival of fun and excitement, as far as I can see. I cannot pinpoint a single cause for distress. You see," she went on, "with older brothers and sisters, there's always something exciting going on and—" She stopped short. "That's it! Jamie is always trying to keep up with the older children. He is forever plotting how not to be left out. *There's* his stress."

"And has he figured out the procedure?"

"Oh, Jamie has a whole bag of tricks. If he wants to participate in a game, first come the promises: 'I *promise* not to cheat the rules' or 'I *promise* I won't be a painy neck'; or if it is a board or a card game that is in question, 'I *promise* I'll a'ways 'member to sit with my legs crossed...like this'—the way he is taught to sit quietly in nursery school. If he cannot think of what else to promise, he falls back on some dim notion of polite behavior: 'I *promise* to 'member to a'ways wash my hands before I play.' Finally, when he has exhausted all his charm and sly cunning, he pulls out his last stop: 'An' if you won't let me play, I won't invite you to my birthday party!' But, once he's allowed to join in their activities, his behavior is irreproachable."

The constitutional picture of *Causticum* was complete.

Ɂ❧

Causticum is most often prescribed for a child's enlarged glands; warts; growing pains; restlessness in the legs at night; the above-mentioned twitchings and jerkings of some part of the body when in bed; rheumatic joint pains, which may well be brought on by exposure to a cold wind; and for coughs with (or from) a tickling in the throat or larynx: incessant, dry, night and day; the child cannot cough deep enough, the expectoration slips back again. *Causticum* is also given for bedwetting (as with *Sepia* often before midnight) or for the spurting of urine from coughing, sneezing, and laughing. Even though good physical coordination (like good mental balance) is more often the norm, occasionally, the remedy is prescribed when isolated groups of muscles are impaired, causing speech defects or poor voice control, poor sphincter control, and muscular disabilities that affect the gross movements (the child is slow learning to walk or is unsteady on his feet) or the finer movements (difficulty in writing out his letters); or the child is simply clumsy in his movements. In terms of the more prominent modalities, wind, cold, drafts, change of weather or extremes of temperature bring on complaints; the child is *better* from warmth, motion (not too strenuous), and, paradoxically, from cold drinks.

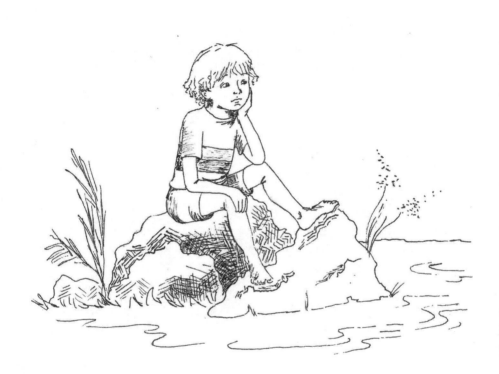

Thuja

(ARBORVITAE)

T*huja* holds a unique position in the gallery of children's archetypes. Quite apart from its own far from simple personality (sometimes gentle, ethereal, otherworldly; at other times harsh, quarrelsome, conniving), in the homoeopathic treatment of children it is the remedy most frequently prescribed "constitutionally" for types other than its own (*Sulphur* and *Tuberculinum* are close contenders). The reasons for this will be examined later in this chapter. Suffice it at this point to recognize the personality picture, which is the same both for inherently *Thuja* children and those who need the remedy due to force of circumstance.

In infancy, the features that stand out and point to the remedy are, first of all, a failure to thrive: poor sleep and poor nursing, often accompanied by much discomfort and crying, as if in protest at landing here on earth. During this stage the child is also distinguished by a fear of and resistance to change. *Thuja* does not respond well to transitions of any kind—either external (a changing environment) or internal (the normal course of growth and development). The infant screams with terror when carried from one room to the next or when transferred from one pair of caring hands to another; later, a change in diet is occasion for stormy weather. Transitions from sleeping to waking and vice versa are other traumas. The child wakens in a grumpy, petulant mood, ready to cry on the slightest pretext, and then is so wired up before nap time or at night that he is unable to get to sleep—the more tired he is, the more resistant. And every new stage of growth (teething, beginning to sit up, to crawl, or to walk) throws him off balance—as is reflected in his disturbed behavior.

The older child exhibits emotional inflexibility. He is disoriented by fluctuations in the family routine (such as someone usurping his favorite seat in the car or at the table), which other siblings accept with equanimity. He displays a temper when forced to switch activities or is interrupted for meals. He refuses to listen to reason when some fixed idea of his is tampered with (such as an article of clothing he has set his mind on wearing or some particular food he has set his mind on eating), regardless of how inappropriate for the occasion. All of this reflects a lack of ease in this world—an inability to go along with the flow of everyday life, with all its setbacks, changes, and variations.

Afflictions reflecting varying degrees of mental confusion, poor social skills, or lack of social awareness (including immature behavior) can also point to *Thuja*. The type becomes too quickly unhinged when excited or tired and is emotionally too labile or easily upset. At times there is a sense of alienation from the world and the rest of humanity, and the child acts as if he is a stranger to the basic skills of life. For instance, in intellectual skills there might be little order or retention. Some days he will know a bit of information; other days he will not. Sometimes he will spell words correctly; at other times not *(Baryta carbonica)*. In talking he might exhibit a rambling style or difficulty finding words. Frequently, long before he has time to finish his thought others will have ceased listening, proceeding on to other topics. Sometimes he makes inappropriate remarks, seemingly irrelevant to the subject at hand (although there does exist a tenuous connection if one takes the trouble to trace the missing links); or, to conceal his awkwardness, he talks a blue streak, often too loudly. In more extreme cases the youngster, feeling different and excluded from this world—and consequently unwanted and unloved—resorts to sobbing and raging. Yet simultaneously he combats with every fiber of his being the assumption of responsibilities appropriate for his age or any discipline that might work to diminish his social ineptness and mental confusion. Additionally, like a premature adolescent, the child mopes discontentedly around the house, unable to amuse himself, constantly seeking distraction but satisfied with none ("I can't stand life. It's so boring. I want to die").

Thuja's unease in, or not quite being of, this world occasionally assumes the form of detachment from reality. The confused, "otherworldly" child lives largely in a realm of his own creative fancy, peopled by imaginary friends, which to him is more real than the world of our five senses. He is not fully present in this world, not fully engaged. For instance, he will sit dreaming in class or at meals, not paying attention to what is going on around him and not responding to direct address. If told to do something, he wanders away and occupies himself with something else. Or, if told *not* to do something (like rock in his chair at the dinner table), he stops, then a moment later

resumes rocking. He does not argue, nor is he actively disobedient, but is inattentive, lost in his own thoughts. Thus, also, at the
end of a car trip, he sits dazed, not moving, still buckled in his
seat belt when all others have gotten out, as if not knowing
what is expected of him. Things seem unfamiliar to him; people
react strangely, incomprehensibly. Living in this reality, he finds
himself experiencing the bewilderment of an Alice in Wonder-
land.

These feelings of foreignness or otherworldliness are manifested in additional ways. Some children will express themselves
in an amusing if not quite correct manner, as if their own language were foreign to them. One five-year-old, envying her
older sister's obvious enjoyment in reading *Little Women,* inquired when would *she* be old enough to read books by Louisa
May Alcohol. Unwelcome serious discussions with her parents
about her behavior she called serious "disgustions," and she
deplored the "locomotion" they created. Another child will talk
like a little old philosopher, seriously and precociously discussing metaphysical subjects such as the afterlife and the existence
of angels or other incarnate spirits. Still another, seemingly attuned to the spirit aspects of nature, will claim to hear voices in
the wind and sea or even the rocks, and to hold conversations
with earth spirits inhabiting the trees, shrubs, flowers, and streams.

Such, for example, was Opal Whiteley, who was born and
reared in a lumber camp in Oregon around the turn of the century and who, between the ages of five and seven, kept a diary
that beautifully captures the ethereal quality of a predominantly
Thuja child:

> I have thinks I was once a tree growing in the forest:
> now all trees are my brothers… I did wonder how I

> would feel if I was a very little piece of wood that got chopped out of a very big tree. I felt of the feelings of the wood. They did have a very sad feel....

And

> Now are come the days of brown leaves....They flutter on the ground. When the brown leaves flutter...they talk with the wind. I hear them tell of their borning days when they did come into the world as leaves...they told how they were part of earth and air before their tree-borning days. And now in gray days of winter they go back to the earth again.*

Children of this ethereal type might display a special way with animals, communicating with them almost as other children communicate with their peers. A literary example is Fodder-wing (from Marjorie Kennan Rawlings's *The Yearling),* the delicate, unworldly child born into a family of burly, rough Florida backwoodsmen, who, to compensate for his physical deformity and a slightly affected mind, develops a fanciful imagination and an uncanny way of befriending the furred and feathered wildlife of the swamps. So strong is his kinship with his natural environment that even after his death, his spirit (as sensed by his friend Jody Baxter) lingers on in the scrub country of the Florida Uplands:

> Something of Fodder-wing had been always where the wild creatures fed and played. Something of him would be always near them. Fodder-wing was like the trees [note the arborvitae]. He was of the earth, as they were earthy, with his gnarled, frail roots in the sand....A part

---

* From *The Diary of Opal Whiteley: Journal of an Understanding Heart.* Boston: The Atlantic Monthly Press, 1920.

of him had been always outside his twisted body. It had come and gone like the wind.

Furthermore, this is the youngster who might actually remember past incarnations, talk with angels, or communicate with the spirits of departed souls. When the grandparents of a girl of eight died in a car accident, for a while afterward she sensed their presence around her during sleep and would pick up messages they were relaying to other members of the family. And subsequently over the years, they would appear to her in premonitory dreams.

Altogether, with *Thuja,* the boundaries between this and other realities can be so fluid that the child is not quite certain to which world he belongs, and he experiences sensations of his mind being separated from his body. In *Ignatia* this feeling is experienced in acute states of shock or grief, but in *Thuja* this sensation is constitutional or chronic. His mind is floating out there in the ozone, while his body is left behind, somewhere on earth.

Complicating the *Thuja* picture are the contradictory aspects of the personality. In the younger child this trait manifests primarily as inconsistencies in likes, dislikes, and desires. One can never anticipate his reaction to any given situation. One time he likes some activity, another time he does not. He begs for a certain food, but as soon as it is prepared, he rejects it. One hour some child is his special friend, another moment he is not; but then an hour later he is welcomed back again into *Thuja*'s good graces. The *Tuberculinum* child, too, is notorious for his contradictory, capricious behavior; but with him it is a passing phase. *Thuja*'s contradictory aspects are the more incomprehensible and unsettling to parents because there is a constant flipping back and forth—or perhaps, more accurately, a *cycling* in his behavior.

The same duality of tastes, preferences, and affections is seen in the older child. For instance, he might entertain a liking for both horror books and movies as well as for refined or even sentimental ones. For friends he chooses both the finest spirits among his peers and, antithetically, the most unruly ones. All openness and affection one moment, he is secretive and unloving the next. Positive and negative emotions seem to contend for supremacy within his soul.

The *Thuja* adolescent is quick to feel estranged from or misunderstood by his family. The instabilities and perturbations of a young soul transiting this particularly stressful passage in human growth is bound to disorient the type that responds adversely to transitions of any kind. Caught up in a web of self-doubt and self-reproach, in emotions that are conflicting or incomprehensible to him, this adolescent needs to prove to himself that he does not belong in this world, and vacillates between feeling either too sensitive and good for it or too awkward and blemished— between feeling insufficiently loved and undeserving of love. Certainly, of efforts at self-control there is little trace, as he gives way to the humor of the moment. And a physical recoil from touch or an irascibility at being addressed go hand-in-hand with an unbounded capacity for taking offense—whether at being noticed *or* ignored, at being either left alone or at *not* being left alone.

Likewise, at this point the *Thuja* perverse sensitivity is amplified: a tendency to be overly sensitive about the wrong things (such as imagined slights) and insensitive about the right ones (the needs and feelings of others). Moreover, like *Natrum muriaticum,* he bitterly resents (and repels) those who are most anxious to help him, precisely because their concern interferes with his feeling of being alienated, unappreciated, and misunderstood. Finally, either he talks at too great length and with too much intensity, without listening to others, or he retires sulky and morose, barring access to his room and avoiding the sight of people.

At this stage, too, many a *Thuja* adolescent likes to live in a state of squalor. In these surroundings he feels more comfortable, since they correspond, on the physical plane, to the disorder in himself. This, to be sure, is also a *Sulphur* characteristic. But while the *Sulphur* adolescent might similarly like squalid disorder, although he similarly abuses his hair and clothes and is possibly even more argumentative, demanding, and utterly selfish, he does not emit that aura of profound emotional *dis*-ease. One recognizes that much of this cloud of adolescence (together with the abuse of hair and dress) will disperse on its own, with time. Lurking in *Thuja's* dark moods, however, is a deeper disturbance of the psyche, which the natural course of things does little to dispel; often it must be consciously addressed with outside guidance and help. In short, when *Thuja* is the underlying picture, the adolescent, with the type's tendency to blow things out of proportion, experiences the familiar traits of feeling wronged, misunderstood, and alienated from and therefore useless in this world to an exponential degree.

And yet, here again, equally to be recognized as *Thuja* is the adolescent who emanates thoughtfulness and a spiritual quality rare for one of his or her age; and whose performance in art, writing, or on a musical instrument carries an inspired, transcendent quality—as if truly coming from another world.

A major factor contributing to the picture of the maladjusted *Thuja* personality is multiple vaccinations at too early an age, before the nervous system has had time to develop. The young child whose psyche is fragile and tenuously balanced to begin with, simply cannot assimilate so many foreign antigens and proteins injected into his bloodstream without the assault causing a major disturbance in the undeveloped nervous system and psyche. Confused as to which cells are unequivocally his own and which are foreign to him, some part of his connection with this world, already too delicate, is ruptured, and his psyche loses touch with accepted reality.

The adverse sequelae of youngsters sensitive to inoculation are multiple. Among the most common physical ones are repeated ear infections; chronic nasal catarrhs (with a tenacious green mucous); diarrhea; eczemas, which when suppressed with medications can develop into asthma; and eating disorders (either poor appetite or, conversely, not knowing when to stop eating). Furthermore, *Thuja* has proved itself invaluable in a number of wide-range neurological disorders, including sleep disturbances, head-banging in infancy and excessive rocking in the older child *(Tuberculinum)*, or seizure activity, with onset traced back to the time of or shortly after inoculation.

The older overvaccinated child might exhibit some loss of emotional or intellectual responsiveness or display diminished social or behavioral awareness. Oblivious to the impression he is producing, in school he acts silly, giggles without cause, makes inappropriate remarks, bothers other children by unwelcome touching or kissing, or in other ways disrupts their work. At home he will rebel against the normal assumption of responsibilities that the maturing process entails, such as attending to the care of his person or his room. The frequency and severity of his oppositional behavior is often quite out of proportion to some simple suggestion or admonition. Additionally, a lack of self-control, combined with restlessness, easy distraction, and an inability to concentrate on the matter at hand, exposes him to the catchall labels of "hyperactivity" or "attention deficit disorder."* Also, many a child diagnosed as dyslexic, dyscalculic, or with some other learning disabilities will require this remedy.

Although *Thuja* plays a prominent role in antidoting the adverse side-effects of vaccination in children, other remedies, such as *Silica, Sulphur, Calcarea carbonica,* and *Natrum muriaticum,* have also proven of value. Nor is inoculation necessarily the sole contributing factor to *Thuja's* untoward behavior and poor social skills, since even unvaccinated children may demonstrate similar behavior. Whatever the cause, over the decades of pediatric practice, *Thuja* has repeatedly displayed a signal capacity to mitigate or cure the imbalances and disorders described above.

≥€

Physically, children requiring *Thuja* might display warts, moles, naevi, or other forms of skin excrescences; tenacious,

---

* When dealing with violent, uncontrolled behavior or more severe emotional derangements, such remedies as *Belladonna* (Deadly nightshade), *Hyoscyamus* (Henbane), *Stramonium* (Thorn apple), *Tarentula hispania* (Spanish spider), or *Veratrum album* (White hellebore) are often called for.

green mucous discharge from the nose; a tendency to eczema which, if suppressed with allopathic medication, can develop into asthma; fungoid growths; brittle, soft, discolored, or deformed nails; forcibly expelled, gurgling, explosive, gushing stool—sometimes solid matter mixed with water; acrid foot sweats; easy decay of teeth.

Among the more prominent modalities are: *worse* around 3:00 a.m.; during the waxing moon; cold damp weather; yearly; and, of course, vaccination; *better* from warm wind and air; wrapping the head; spiritual help or guidance; healing touch.

Stramonium

(Thorn apple)

Stramonium, best known for its power to heal *Belladonna*-like deliriums and cerebral disturbances, also possesses a constitutional aspect to its picture. From an early age, the child displays signs of feeling at odds with his environment. There is an agitation and unease about him, also erratic changes of mood and behavior, that foreshadow the difficulties he will experience later accommodating to this world.

He is not a robust or buoyant or happy child, which is at times reflected in his very looks: a pallid complexion, wrinkled forehead, troubled eyes, and an expression haggard beyond his years. Because of an innate suspiciousness of humanity and the world he lives in, he acts timid with most people and is chronically apprehensive, as if expecting the worst to befall him. When, occasionally, the child is robust and buoyant, happy and bold, there is an unsettled, unquiet, excessive quality to these desirable traits.

Much of the time he truly is suffering—although not so much from physical pain. In fact, the type can be remarkably insensitive to pain. If, in a temper or passion, the youngster knocks himself against the corner of a table, bangs his head on a hard object, or cuts himself with a sharp utensil, he hardly seems to be aware of the injury; the older child who, in his frustration, punches his hand through a wall, hardly seems to feel it. It is in spirit that he suffers. In contrast, the *Tuberculinums* or *Nux vomicas* are seldom equally tormented by their temper tantrums or the disruptive side of their natures. *Others* suffer when they start acting out, but not they themselves. But the *Stramonium* child who bites or kicks in anger, or screams as if beside himself and strikes out at others, is striking out at an intolerable world.

Intolerable to him because, apart from an inharmonious disposition, his whole nervous system is off-kilter. On the one hand, he is easily enervated by bright light, everyday sounds (such as running water) or social contact ("Go away! Leave me alone!" he snarls in a burst of irritability which he seldom scruples to control). Yet on the other hand, he is afraid of silence and solitude (to combat which he may constantly demand special attention) and dreads the dark. This is one of the types that suffers from "seasonal affective disorder," displaying a marked deterioration in behavioral patterns after the fall equinox and during dark, cloudy days.

There exists, to be sure, a sweet, affectionate side to *Stramonium*, as well. Beneath the surface disharmony, he harbors strong loyalties, is deeply attached to one particular sibling or to one or both parents and, when older, will frequently possess a healthy, bantering relationship with them. ("I know that I come from a family where no member ever admits to being wrong," an eleven-year-old declared. "So my genes are insisting that this time *I* get my own way.") He seldom suffers from lack of generosity and is a sensitive, reliable friend.

As with *Lachesis,* the nature appears to be conflicted. In the *Lachesis* child, however, the struggles of conscience between right and wrong are only sporadic. Most of the time he is energetically pursuing a full and active life, and his moral conflicts do not affect his vital, creative personality. *Stramonium* is different. Despite unmistakable signs of being gifted in some particular field, the child's continuous inner conflicts impede a full or satisfying existence, and his precocity is offset by a perverse willfulness. More similar in *gestalt* to the conflicted *Thuja,* a struggle as to whether benign or malignant emotions will possess his soul keeps him in a chronic state of anxiety, ill-ease, and guilt. Guilt then induces low self-esteem (this last is, in part, why he bursts into vehement sobs when contradicted or reprimanded), which in turn makes him feel unhappy and misunderstood. Unhappiness drives him to frequent altercations with siblings or parents, to behave rudely or in some socially unacceptable manner, and there may even be violence in his behavior, as he attempts to make others and the world dance to his tune. All this brings on more guilt and anxiety, as he gets caught in a vicious circle from which he finds it hard to extricate himself.

However, *Stramonium* as a rule is not as ethereal or otherworldly as *Thuja* can be—not as dissociated from his body, and from reality. Although uncomfortably so, he is more present in this world. But he can exhibit the same lack of responsiveness. The child is told to do something—as, for instance, get dressed for school—and half an hour later he is still wandering around in his pajamas, with a sock in his hand. There may also be some mental confusion. The child does not answer questions, complete sentences, or find the right words; or there is an

inability to concentrate or focus on schoolwork, and he may
have difficulty sticking with one idea. Or, similar to both *Thuja*
and *Natrum muriaticum, Stramonium* suddenly becomes loquacious; and, seemingly driven by some uncontrollable force,
talks at too great length, not sensing when to stop.

The adolescent feels, and often *is,* different from his peers.
He has an original mind, might possess a quirky sense of humor, and continues to be strongly attached and loyal to certain
family members or to a friend. But often these positive characteristics are undermined by an obstinate, headstrong nature and
a tendency to be sulky or engage in senseless arguments or
quarreling.

Certainly, *Stramonium* wants to be liked and tries to behave well. It is just that he too easily "loses it" and is unable to
control himself—a factor that contributes to his social and moral
unease.

ॐ

Since "the entire force of this drug seems to be expanded
on the brain" (Boericke),* and the remedy is administered to
children almost exclusively for learning or behavioral disorders
and poor social skills, other than awakening terrified from sleep,
sometimes screaming with fright, or experiencing choreic symptoms or convulsions of isolated groups of muscles, there are no
noteworthy physical symptoms in the *Stramonium* child's archetypal picture.

---

* See Suggested Readings.

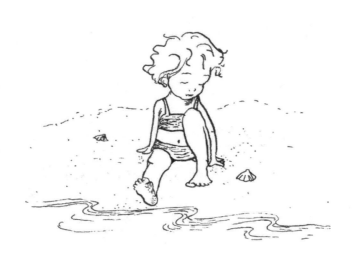

Silica

(PURE FLINT)

I n children, the *Silica* archetype partakes generously of the natures of *Pulsatilla* and *Calcarea carbonica*. This does not, however, preclude the remedy's possessing a personality picture distinctly its own.

Silica's affinity with *Pulsatilla* is particularly observed in the younger child's shyness and fear of strangers, his clinging manner when ailing, and a tendency to cry easily from hurt feelings or a rebuke. Also, being neither of an aggressive nor of an overly assertive disposition, he is more likely to retire from a hostile or difficult situation than to fight it. But although at first glance the type displays the *Pulsatilla* mildness and docility, in reality he is not as malleable and yielding or as susceptible to outside influence. Diffident and self-effacing he may be, and shrinking from making waves, but he does not allow himself to be imposed on. Nor is he irresolute; once he arrives at a decision or conviction, he holds to it, in contrast to *Pulsatilla*'s frequent fluctuations.

When it comes to the question of independence, *Silica* more closely resembles *Calcarea carbonica*. Not only does the child have a mind of his own, but also, by being unrelenting and wearing down another's resistance, he eventually induces others to consider his wishes and deal with him on his own terms. Thus, the older child who dislikes his boarding school, yet cannot persuade his parents to bring him home or send him elsewhere, begins to apply methods of passive persuasion, such as not answering his parents' letters and refusing to telephone them. Instead of resorting to active misbehavior (as would *Sulphur* or *Nux vomica),* he carries his point by developing elusive complaints or a malingering attitude. Like *Calcarea carbonica,* then, tenacity and persistence are more often *Silica's* style: his obstinacy taking the form of stubborn resistance or *refusal* to act, rather than a bullheaded insistence on acting unreasonably.

Like *Calcarea,* too, *Silica* can be excessively attached to the home. The remedy, especially when prescribed preventively, has benefitted any number of homesick children. A case in point was the ten-year-old boy who would call his parents from summer camp every morning at 6:00 a.m. and tearfully beg to return home. The family situation made this impossible, so his harassed mother would try to persuade him to "stick it out like a man." The conversations would then run along the following philosophical lines:

"Why should I stick it out? Will I be *less* of a man if I don't?"

"Well, not exactly—but summer camp is part of your educational experience."

"How can it be an educational experience when I am so unhappy?"

"Even unhappiness is an integral part of being alive."

"But why *should* unhappiness be a part of being alive?"

The best the mother could think of was, "That's the way life is. That's one of life's lessons."

"But do you *want* me to be unhappy when I'm still so young? *Please,* can't I learn this lesson later when I'm a little older?"

Ignatia for the acute condition (see that chapter) helped the boy to overcome his homesickness at the time. But it was *Silica,* prescribed constitutionally prior to leaving home, that assisted him during the following two summers, so that no *Ignatia* was required.

Even though the *Silica* child might be physically delicate and emotionally sensitive, the psyche is stable. He is even-tempered, reliable, free from boastfulness or desire for display. There is nothing of the bully about him and seldom does he feel compelled to assert his will by overtly dominating others. And no type, not even *Arsenicum album,* is more conscientious; no child cleans up his desk more meticulously in school or is more scrupulous in caring for a younger sibling at home, even when intimidated by the responsibility. (One five-year-old girl, while competently, conscientiously helping to care for her six-month-old sister, was in such awe of the baby's commanding gestures and imperious grunts, that she appealed to her mother, "Mommy, tell Jennie to stop bossing me around!") Later, the *Silica* student will, with the same diligence, dedicate himself to his studies, even if feeling overwhelmed by the work required. In fact, the "eternal student" who haunts the university libraries and classrooms, year after year, because he never feels sufficiently prepared to complete his studies, is frequently a *Silica.*

And he does easily feel overwhelmed; the nature is a timorous as well as cautious one. Too often, for him, the risks of an enterprise seem to outweigh the advantages. The younger child cannot bring himself to attempt some feat in gym class or on the playground that his peers perform without turning a hair; or he will only ride his new bicycle alone in his yard or on the back patio, not with his peers on a safe street or in the park, for fear of an ignominious fall in public. The older child often lacks confidence in school. Although his skills are good and he knows the material well, he still sits quietly at the back of the classroom, seldom volunteering to answer questions and hoping that the teacher will not remember to call on him. This contrasts with the self-assured *Sulphur,* who loves being called on and is always raising his hand (whether or not he knows the right answer) as well as with *Arsenicum album* and *Nux vomica* who are also eager to answer in class—and usually answer correctly. In general, *Silica,* averse to being noticed, will go to great lengths to avoid attention.

With the passage of time, the older child grows discriminating, exacting, somewhat critical—not so much faultfinding as selective in his judgment and fastidious in his tastes. Certainly, he can be difficult to please. Even in such a trifling matter as approving of a pair of socks, *Silica* can display extreme fastidiousness ("They crinkle up in my shoes, at the toes"; "The cotton is too stiff"; "The nylon in them makes them too hot"; "They slouch at the ankles"; "They're too tight at the ankles"; "It's the right color, but too shiny"; and so forth). And a clothes tag rubbing against the skin or sleeping on a wrinkled sheet is intolerable. Here *Silica* is reminiscent of the overrefined princess in the fairytale who could not sleep because of the one pea under her many mattresses. Reminiscent, too, of the princess is the type's frequently encountered emotional refinement. This last may manifest as stoicism in the face of adversity, reticence as to his or her own disappointments or desires in consideration for others' feelings, and a scrupulous honesty.

These characteristics set the child somewhat apart from others and he may grow detached. To guard his sensitive nature against injury, he begins to dissociate from the intrusive, unattractive aspects of this world as well as from too intense emotions, such as entanglements in family disputes or peer relationships. Even in friendship he is reserved rather than outgoing. This trait might well make him appear aloof, standoffish, or even selfish. But he does not wish to snub, judge, or hurt people; he merely wishes to be left alone.

It is, in fact, precisely because it takes this sensitive child a long time to recover from emotional disharmony that he develops, then cultivates, the self-protective techniques of self-effacement, imperturbability, detachment, and a low-key self-sufficiency. Curiously, the type's slow recuperative powers on the mental-emotional plane find their physical counterpart in the slow healing of a variety of ailments, especially skin complaints: the unending suppuration of surface injuries, infections and fissures; festering of splinters and of the skin round the nails; boils and abscesses that refuse to come to a head; ulcerous infections that do not heal; and the like.

❧

The physical overlap between *Silica* and *Pulsatilla* is encountered in such childhood ailments as enuresis, coughs, colds, ear infections (*Silica* is rich in ear symptoms, such as catarrhs, blockages, draining, hearing loss, abnormal noises, rupture of the drum, etc.); and, in general, this remedy often works when *Pulsatilla* is unavailing.

The even more pervasive overlap between *Silica* and

Calcarea carbonica calls for a comparative and differential analysis of their respective pictures. Both types might possess big heads and protruding abdomens (shaped like inverted saucers) and manifestly lax muscle tone. The younger children might be slow learning to sit up, stand up, or walk, and show little inclination to try. While the *Calcarea carbonica* child is more obviously "floppy," *Silica* can be equally flexible and rubbery—to the extent that the young pianist's or violinist's career is handicapped by fingers that are too flexible and collapsing, while the young gymnast's muscular control is inhibited by excessive elasticity. Both types are easily fatigued and perspire freely around the head and neck, particularly during sleep; but with *Silica* one encounters, additionally, offensive excoriating foot sweats that can eat through socks and shoe leather. Both types can be milk intolerant, developing diarrhea or vomiting it, and occasionally even mother's milk disagrees. But *Silica* exhibits more signs of malnutrition or poor assimilation of food and might look emaciated *(Calcarea,* as noted earlier, looks well-nourished). Either remedy can be given preventively for recurring sore throats that settle in the tonsils or glands of the neck and for children with repeated ear infections. Both types are sensitive to cold in every form; but *Silica* is especially so to drafts to the head, to cool bathing after becoming heated, and to air conditioning. Finally, both types are affected by the stages of the moon; however, whereas *Calcarea* is aggravated primarily during the full moon, *Silica*'s aggravations are primarily during the new moon.

Not infrequently, the two types can be distinguished by their weight, build, and physical appearance. The *Calcarea carbonica* child is usually heavy, flabby, phlegmatic, and with full or rosy cheeks, while *Silica* is of slighter build, with small, regular features and fine veins showing through the clear, nearly translucent skin; often pale and sometimes puny, with a pinched, wizened, "old" look.

When blonde, *Silica* is more truly blond than *Calcarea carbonica* in the sense that the fine, often thin, wispy hair remains fair and silky-textured into adulthood. This combination of wispy blonde hair, delicate frame and features, and alabaster skin often combine to make the *Silica* child appear too angelic for this world.

Baryta carbonica

(CARBONATE OF BARYTA)

Baryta carbonica is often prescribed for children who present a mental-emotional picture of failure to thrive. Lack of self-confidence, an excessive fearfulness in social situations, weak concentration powers (one day the child will remember how to spell a word or do a sum, another day not), or delayed skills in intellectual development are among the most prominent guiding symptoms. Altogether, the diffident, insecure nature is reminiscent of a snail that ventures to protrude its head only a little way out of its shell, then shrinks back at the first hint of a threat.

Baryta carbonica perceives anything that infringes on the familiar or the routine or confronts him with a challenge (even if quite appropriate to his age) as a threat. The young child dreads attending nursery school or even going to a party for fear he will encounter children who might tease, criticize, or talk about him behind his back. Like *Calcarea carbonica*, sensing that he is not as quick or articulate as his peers, he is all apprehension; and even if others are laughing *with* and not *at* him, he fears he is being ridiculed (whereas a *Sulphur* or a *Phosphorus* loves the attention of being teased and joins in the laughter). One little *Baryta carbonica* girl was asked why she did not enjoy school. Did she not like her kind teacher and her classmates? And why wouldn't she participate more in class or join in the children's games? She replied, "Sure, I like 'em. But I'm always afraid that they'll laugh at me. And then I feel like they've stepped on me and *squashed* me, like an aluminum can."

As a consequence of such sensitivities, the *Baryta* child might withdraw into himself and refuse even to try to mix or actively participate. When in a group, he sits quietly observing, taking in what is going on around him but, fearing a social blunder, giving out little himself. Or he remains wrapped in his own thoughts, oblivious to his surroundings, and altogether relying on his own resources for entertainment. At times, like *Thuja,* he loses himself in his own fantasy world, inventing imaginary friends for companions or stories that run on from day to day, to the point where he might start to act somewhat "out of it," and find himself isolated.

Yet such behavior need not necessarily denote mental backwardness. It is more a *Calcarea*-like resistance to being saddled with responsibilities not to his liking or to being forced into some uncongenial mold. *Baryta carbonica* simply has his own approach to the world, his own mode of behavior. For instance, he might exhibit a quaint, old-fashioned manner, as did the six-year-old who was captivated by an (admittedly enchanting) prima ballerina in her twenties who lived across the street. From time to time he would telephone her and say, "You go up to your bathroom on the second floor and look out the window, and I'll go up to my bathroom on the second floor and look out the window, and then we'll wave to each other." Or he can be surprisingly New Age. When he was asked what he wanted as a present for his seventh birthday, one *Baryta* youngster replied that he wished for a series of body massages with a masseuse who was a family friend.

Occasionally, the child comes out with meditative or original remarks that are thoughtful beyond his years. A five-year-old girl was out on a nature walk with her class.

"Look there, to the horizon, where the trees are touching the sky," her teacher pointed out. "Aren't they beautiful!"

"*Are* the trees touching the sky?" the girl inquired.

"Why, yes, don't you see?"

There was a long silence. Then, "I'm looking an' looking, but *still* I don't understand," was the unexpected response.

Or when pondering death, she asked her mother, "After death, do people smile?"

"Oh, yes," she was assured. "Death is merely the beginning of a new and often wonderful life."

"But can the people who *stay behind* still smile?" the little girl persisted.

The snail-like mentality can be observed in the older child who not only is without undo pretensions as to his own capacities but, like *Silica,* feels thoroughly uncomfortable in the limelight, even when it is deserved. For this, as well as the reasons mentioned above, he might shy away from group activities or too much socializing with his peers. And the overall picture brings to mind the words of American essayist and poet James Russell Lowell: "Solitude is useful for the imagination as society is wholesome for the character." *Baryta carbonica* has a healthy imagination but could profit, one feels, from some salutary peer society.

The older *Baryta* child might grow more socially inclined, but then another difficulty arises; he is too apt to view himself as a weak character. This label conveniently absolves him from having to be conscientious about schoolwork, adhere to sound resolutions, and assume tedious responsibilities. Such a fatalistic (not to say defeatist) attitude renders him somewhat akin to the indolent *Calcarea carbonica,* with whom he shares the philosophy, "Why do today what can be put off until tomorrow?" In contrast to *Silica* who, while suffering from an equal lack of self-confidence, still perseveres (and succeeds), *Baryta carbonica* decides that there is no point in opposing the decrees of Destiny and allows himself to sink into intellectual idleness and poor performance in school while pursuing an active social life. It is as if he has not the physical or moral strength to attend to both peer society and his mental development.

⅍

In *Baryta carbonica's* physical picture, too, there can be a failure to thrive. Poor appetite or poor sleep, low vital energy, stunted growth, a susceptibility to upper respiratory and chest infections, eye infections, ear infections, or swollen tonsils and glands are all encountered in the child in need of this remedy, indicating this remedy's close physical relationship with *Calcarea carbonica* and *Silica.* (For more detail, see the chapters on *Baryta carbonica's* better-known "siblings.")

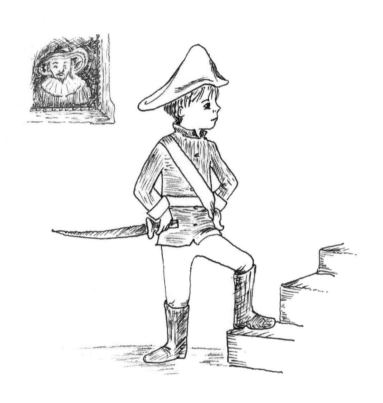

Nux vomica[§]

(POISON NUT)

Nux vomica presents an interesting combination of *Sulphur* and *Arsenicum album*. Like *Sulphur,* the child is energetic, self-reliant, enterprising, and makes his presence felt. Like *Arsenicum*, he is competent, intense, and anxiety-prone. The easy irritability, overexcitation, and uneven temper are, however, entirely his own.

Nux vomica is usually the possessor of a good mind. Some specific type of cleverness is encountered even in the very young. For instance, one four-year-old, a precocious speller, would, when not feeling well at night, cry out imperiously, "M-O-M, get me N-U-X!" The older child, in his intellectual restlessness, develops a wide range of interests and skills. He is ambitious, highly competitive, and determined to succeed (even if sometimes unobtrusively so). From an early age he fosters the conviction that application and hard work bring success and then acts on this conviction. Often he is a perfectionist and displays an *Arsenicum*-like love for order, neatness, and methodicalness. He also displays a fine capacity to think things through to his

157

own advantage and is highly conscious of power. Boys who are fascinated with books on warfare and the lives of famous emperors, kings, generals, or others wielding power, and who from a tender age begin to devour books on World Wars I and II, are often found to be *Nux vomicas* or *Sulphurs*. *Arsenicum* makes as good a commanding general in everyday life, but in youth he is less interested in actual warfare.

Similar to *Arsenicum album*, *Nux* can be a highly controlling individual. Given the chance, the boy will take over and begin to dictate others' lives. When he plays board games, he corrects his opponent at checkers or chess; when he is on the playing field, he shouts out commands to his teammates. (*Sulphur* simply goes his own way, *expecting* others to follow.) The girl equally loves to give advice (often unsolicited) and is ever eager to assume the responsibility of class president or some other position of authority. Furthermore, fastidious to the point of faultfinding, the young *Nux* is often critical of another's manners and performance and exhibits anxiety when things are not done in what he deems the right way. For instance, he becomes annoyed at a peer's sloppy performance in school ("If he doesn't know the answer, he shouldn't raise his hand!") or at a recital ("Why does he decide to play a piece obviously too difficult for him, and then mess it up!") Or an eight-year-old will rebuke a parent: "Yes, you had the right to ask my friend to help with the dishes, but you didn't ask him in the right way. You must be more tactful and less direct about it." The child is all the more sensitive about his friend's feelings because he himself is exceedingly sensitive to criticism and disrespect. His pride being easily wounded, he is touchy and prickly, quick to feel attacked and to bristle into instant self-defense.

At times, *Nux vomica* exhibits an unexpected considerateness in social situations. If there is not enough of a tasty dish to go around for seconds, similar to *Pulsatilla,* he might forgo his share. Or if there is not sufficient room for a group of boys to fit onto a high platform the better to watch a school game, *Nux* might be the one to step down from this superior vantage point to make way for others. Such behavior is a manifestation of maturity as well as mental refinement, and often the type displays a further maturity in his good understanding of his own nature and his striving for self-improvement.

Because of his tenuous emotional balance and low tolerance for vexations and frustration, self-improvement is by no means an easy undertaking. The child has to truly exert himself to control his testy, hypersensitive disposition and too easily frazzled nerves—not to mention his penchant for hysteria when he is crossed or his desires are thwarted. One twelve-year-old, of an obviously excitable disposition, displayed remarkable self-control at home and school. Although entering adolescence, he never lost his temper, never raised his voice, and seldom allowed himself to become excited over household disagreements or troubles at school. When asked one day if he ever felt anger or frustration, he replied that of course he did, but that having once, in fifth grade, become enraged at a teacher—to the point of wanting to *kill* him—he was subsequently so ashamed of making a spectacle of himself, so appalled at his loss of dignity (observe the *Nux* sensitive pride), that he vowed then and there never again to "spazz out" (a term particularly suitable to *Nux)* and always stay "mellow."

By contrast, there is the *Nux vomica* picture of unruliness—in the individual whose Achilles heel is his unstable temper which he makes no effort to curb. He seems to combine both *Sulphur's* short fuse and *Tuberculinum's* violent, uncontrolled behavior. Not only does the youngster wake up in the morning cross, irritable, or crying, remaining malcontent throughout the day, but more severely, he throws tantrums: yelling wildly, throwing himself down on the ground, smashing his toys, striking out at those trying to calm him, and kicking and biting those attempting to discipline him. The older child is disputatious to an extreme: quick to justify his own mistakes by blaming others, willing—even eager—to enter into combat with whoever thwarts him. He is defiant, always causing reactions, with a tendency continually to test the patience of those in authority. He can be as willful as *Sulphur,* as determined to achieve his ends as *Arsenicum album,* and, like *Medorrhinum,* does not know when to stop—pushing others to the point where he is bound to encounter angry opposition. Later, he might develop into that special breed of contentious adolescent who likes to try out how much he can get away with and provoke conflict in all situations. Not for him is the passive resistance of a *Calcarea carbonica* or the pertinacity of a *Silica;* similar to *Sulphur* and *Medorrhinum, Nux* in his rebelliousness actively seeks confrontation.

The adolescent *Nux* girl's style of discontent is more one of nervous irritability, irascibility, and uncertain moods. She is not as ungovernable as the boy and has better control over her temper, but is easily enervated by an inimical environment. This is the type that becomes exceedingly irritated by music played too loudly or even someone chewing gum too visibly. She is *Arsenicum*-critical of family, friends, and of her own as well as others' performance. Certainly, she is as difficult to please as her male counterpart. Everything must be exactly according to her fastidious tastes and wishes before she can rest easy or allow others to rest easy, as she attempts to govern every aspect of her life and environment. To this end, she might, once again like *Arsenicum album,* become anorexic or bulimic. The condition stems from a similar need to be in complete control of her physique and pride in her superior ability to limit her food intake, rather than from any deep-seated unhappiness or overt mental imbalance. Also, because of her fastidious nature, she may well develop a cliquish attitude in school or other peer environments. Only those of superior refinement or intellect are permitted into her elite circle; the duller, clumsier elements of humanity are excluded.

There is much inherent pride in the girl but, as with the boy, she is willing to work on curbing whatever is defective in her disposition. "Yes, I have a lot of pride," one thirteen-year-old conceded when she was asked to swallow it for the sake of family peace. "But, well...I guess I *can* bring myself to sacrifice a little of it, and go ahead and apologize to Aunt 'Liza. Okay, I'll swallow some of my pride. After all, there's always plenty more where it comes from."

Furthermore, *Nux vomica* can display a *Silica*-like delicacy of scruples as well as the same sweetness of disposition as *Pulsatilla*—even if the latter's gentleness and docility are lacking. The girl will spontaneously offer to prepare a meal or care for a younger sibling if her mother feels unwell and, naturally, does a good job of it. These attractive attributes, when combined with a desire for self-improvement, contribute to that special moral refinement which is encountered both in boys and girls of this constitutional type.

ౚ

With regard to physical symptoms and modalities, *Nux vomica* is prescribed for ailments of the respiratory tract: head colds with much sneezing, spasmodic coughs, seasonal and environmental allergies, asthma; also for ailments of the digestive system, including stomach and abdominal pains, nausea (with inability to vomit), vomiting, diarrhea, and the type's own peculiar form of constipation: ineffectual urging or with an incomplete or unsatisfactory feeling after stool.

This remedy is also called for in extreme sensitivities to the environment. The slightest noises affect the concentration, and his sleep can be disturbed by even a fly in the room; the eyes are sensitive to bright light and sunshine; strong odors give him headaches; and he may be sensitive to cold in every form—the corollary to which is: *better* from wrapping up warm, especially the head, hot drinks and warm food, warm weather. Finally, the child can suffer from insomnia due to disturbing ideas crowding the mind; he has low energy or is in poor spirits in the morning and feels better in the evening, often displaying night energy.

Ignatia

(ST. IGNATIUS BEAN)

T he *Ignatia* constitutional type tends to be nervy, easily excited, quick in perception and, once decided on
some course of action, rapid in execution. Emotionally sensitive to the point of fragility, the child can become ill
from disappointment, frustration, or a mere reprimand. He, or
more especially she, will sob uncontrollably when told, for instance, that she is acting selfish. "I'm not selfish! I'm not! Don't
say I'm selfish! I'm *not!*" she reiterates. And her heartbroken
sobs or even animal-like howls are extremely difficult to quiet.

The child also falls apart when not performing up to expectations—her own or another's. This is the bright girl who is
doing well enough in school, but is feeling the strain. Too many
demands are made on her; or she immerses herself too deeply
in her studies or in practicing a musical instrument, pushing
herself to excel. From this pressure she develops headaches,
tension in the facial muscles, or even tics. She cries too easily
and, with time, she may not be able to function at all.

Typical here was the high-strung girl of twelve who had not

been placed in the honors section of her class. Expectations of high performance had been cultivated both by her parents and by herself, so she felt mortified and began to feel an aversion to everything connected with her school; even her appetite began to decline. Shortly after she was prescribed *Ignatia,* she volunteered, "You know, I'm really glad I didn't make the fast track in school. Now I have more time for extracurricular activities. I've signed up for both drama and glee clubs, and I think I'm going to love them!" Thus, instead of brooding on her failure (and perhaps developing a *Natrum muriaticum* grievance for life, as a result), or losing self-confidence *(Silica)* and refusing in the future to try again *(Calcarea carbonica), Ignatia* helped her cheerfully to go on to something else.

But more frequently, *Ignatia* is prescribed for specific emotional states, regardless of a child's basic constitutional type. It is the preferred remedy for a wide range of emotional imbalances arising from loss, sorrow, unfulfilled longing, or the shattering of some cherished hope—playing a vital role in assisting a child to accept the undesirable but inescapable realities of this world.

Sometimes the child will present the previously described picture of stormy grief. At other times the young sufferer is undemonstrative in sorrow but goes into a gradual decline. Such was the toddler who suddenly began to refuse all food, even milk, and for two months subsisted solely on apple juice. Otherwise she was well-behaved and cheerful, with nothing apparently upsetting her, and the parents were at their wits' end to know what to do: "How *does* one force an eighteen-month-old to eat? You can't reason with her or bribe her, or force food down her throat as if she were a Strasburg goose." Closer inquiry revealed that she had a younger brother and, although she exhibited none of the classic signs of sibling jealousy (nothing but fondness and affection for him), there was the possibility that she was feeling the loss of parental love. A high potency of *Ignatia* was prescribed, once a day for three days. After the first dose she asked for milk; after the second she could be persuaded to eat a dollop of creamed chicken (her favorite food); and after the third, her appetite continued to picked up bit-by-bit, until she was eventually eating normally.

An instance of *articulated Ignatia* sorrow and chagrin at the arrival of a newcomer into the family was the three-year-old who kept insisting that her parents return her baby sister "to Bloomingdale's." She clung to the conviction that new babies came from a department store, despite her parents' more accurate explanations. To their appeal, "How can we let this weak, helpless, thin little creature, who can't even stand up by herself, be sent back where she came from?" the precocious little girl sobbingly pleaded, "Please, why don't you just *try* standing her up on her weak, helpless, skinny little legs, and just *see* if she won't walk back to Bloomingdale's!" Had the child been more aggressively jealous, with a desire to injure the baby, *Lachesis* would have been the preferred remedy.

Another *Ignatia*-requiring situation is homesickness, as was perceived in the case of the ten-year-old *Silica* boy at camp, who begged his mother to please let him come home (see the *Silica* chapter). The hardhearted mother sent her son some *Ignatia* instead, to be taken twice a day until he felt better. After several days there were no more pathetic phone calls and the parents received a bracing postcard: "The food here is wonderful, the activities are just great, and my cabin leader is a *real* neat guy!"

The loss of a beloved pet is yet another situation that commonly calls for *Ignatia*. The remedy possesses a remarkable capacity to attenuate the grieving, and help the young mourner come to terms with irretrievable loss. Equally important, it assists in preventing certain children from morbidly dwelling on some tragic aspects of life, such as the often insensitive or cruel treatment of animals.

Occasionally, in instances of severe grief, the type experiences the sensation of disorientation or dissociation. The child goes about dazed, bewildered, even stupefied. This can be accompanied by lightheadedness, a floating sensation, or blank staring; more seriously, he lapses into a catatonic state. In the same way that nerves are momentarily numbed after the shock of great pain, so the *Ignatia* mental anguish is temporarily numbed by dissociation.

One feature peculiar to the remedy picture is the way in which, with the stabilizing, integrating factor of the personality weakened by trauma and excess emotion, the *Ignatia*-requiring child might begin to embrace the more unhealthy characteristics of several constitutional types simultaneously: *Nux vomica's* irritable sensitivity, nervous irascibility, fault-finding attitude, quarrelsomeness, and readiness to accuse others; *Lycopodium's* dictatorial and autocratic behavior during illness; *Arsenicum's* panicky reaction to not feeling well, critical, demanding nature, and constant complaining; *Pulsatilla's* clinging dependence, weepiness, plaintiveness, and insatiable need for sympathy; *Sepia's* discontent, dissatisfaction with those trying to help, and intolerance of contradiction; the *Phosphorus* lack of emotional restraint, unexpected ingratitude, and collapse into despair when life does not measure up to some romantic ideal; the uncontrolled loquacity and jealous suspiciousness of *Lachesis;* the *Sulphur* explosiveness; the *Tuberculinum* capriciousness and changeable moods; the *Natrum muriaticum* unappeasable anger and resentment, and insistence on dwelling on sad or painful thoughts; and others.

All of this constitutes a formula for hysteria—for which *Ignatia* is one of the principal remedies. And this picture of being caught in a maelstrom of overlapping constitutional pictures, unexpected, conflicting emotions, and confused, contradictory moods is, curiously, paralleled on the physical plane. Thus, in the *Ignatia* patient one encounters the following paradoxes:

- a craving for fresh air, yet being irritated by a breeze,
- during a headache the head feels hot, but amelioration comes from hot, not cold, applications,
- a headache or earache ameliorated by music, not by quiet,
- a toothache relieved by chewing,
- a tickling or spasm in the throat not relieved by coughing—instead a paroxysm of unarrestable coughing is triggered, and the more he coughs, the more he has to cough,
- a pain in the abdomen, side, back, or head relieved (instead of being aggravated) by coughing,
- an empty, feeling in the stomach not relieved or ameliorated by eating,
- when the stomach is upset, the child craves and can tolerate rich cream sauces or indigestible foods and is worse from bland foods such as milk, porridge, toast, or fruit, even while craving them,
- nausea with inability to vomit ameliorated by eating,

- painful or sensitive or swollen areas of the body are better, not worse, from hard pressure,

- the skin itches without any eruption *(Arsenicum),*

- during a fever the child is pale and thirstless, feels chilled, and wants to be covered, while during a chill the face is red, he feels thirsty, and he wants to be uncovered

- there is external coldness together with internal heat,

- an amelioration of painful symptoms from vigorous exercise *(Sepia);*

- and so on, *ad infinitum.*

ॐ

Additional physical symptoms encountered in *Ignatia* are an extreme *Nux vomica*-like sensitivity to noise—the child can be an inordinately light sleeper, wakened by any noise, and when concentrating on mental work, disturbed by the slightest sound. There is an equal sensitivity to odors: to the smell of flowers, perfume, coffee, tobacco; and an intolerance of lack of air in crowded places, elevators, stuffy rooms. Any of these latter conditions can bring on feelings of suffocation or a near-hysterical craving for air.

Carcinosin

E ven though in a child's physical complaints the principal indication for *Carcinosin* (prepared from cancer cell tissue) is a strong family history of cancer (in which case the mental-emotional symptoms described below are of secondary importance), there does exist a *Carcinosin* personality picture, which most closely resembles *Arsenicum album* and *Natrum muriaticum*.

The type often has difficulty dealing with authority; he either subjects himself too obediently to some strong authority or too insistently takes charge himself. This issue might have its roots in excessive parental control; the child strives to live up to certain moral or intellectual demands placed on him and feels culpable when he cannot do so. But the submission he displays is not his true nature—and later he will react to even reasonable authority with too much aggression. On the other hand, there need not be any such a history. With his own critical nature and *Arsenicum*-like desire for high accomplishment and determination to excel, the ambitious *Carcinosin* is quite capable of driv-

ing himself to take on more than he can comfortably (or health-
ily) handle.

Illustrating this characteristic was the exceptionally conscientious high school student who was prescribed the seemingly
obvious "similar remedy," *Arsenicum album,* for his asthma,
with no results whatsoever. Only at the second office visit was it
ascertained that his worst time was not the *Arsenicum* one,
around and after midnight, but after school between 3:30 and
6:30 p.m. The boy's family and the physician thought, at first,
that it was the intense school curriculum as well as athletics that
caused the aggravations. Perhaps these contributed. Even on
weekends and holidays, however, he seemed to be worse at
that time. *Carcinosin* exhibits a 1:00 to 6:00 p.m. aggravation
time and the remedy was accordingly administered—with success.

At times, the young *Carcinosin*'s strong self-motivation develops into an *Arsenicum*-like obsessive-compulsive streak. One
child *must* tie four or five knots in his shoelaces to feel secure in
his sneakers; another fearing contamination, *insistently* washes
(several times) the already clean plate and cup he will be using
at meals; a third, to satisfy the type's self-critical vein and fastidious taste, is *compelled* to go over a penmanship assignment in
school so many times that it ends up looking worse and worse.
And all the while he grows more and more frantic at his failure
to achieve.

Like *Natrum muriaticum,* the *Carcinosin* youngster might
present the picture of confusion and distress at the discrepancy
between the moral principles taught him (tolerance, kindness,
truthfulness) and the inevitable lapses in the daily lives of the
authority figures who guide him. And the older child exhibits

more than a trace of *Natrum muriaticum*'s earnest, dutiful nature, which regards life as a series of hurdles to be surmounted
and hardships to be endured; for which reason he imposes on
himself ethical strictures and then adheres to them through thick
and thin.

A teenage girl was suffering from lingering mononucleosis.
She was of a thoughtful disposition, ultra-aware of the perilous
state of the planet and of man's exploitation of it—and trying to
live in a way commensurate with this awareness. As a result,
she often found herself depressed and wondering whether there
was any meaning to life. These heavy feelings (together with
her physical complaints of headaches and fatigue) she kept largely
to herself, shunning attempts at sympathy and rejecting outside
assistance. Yet all the while she was seeking approval for her
elevated moral standards and was aggrieved at not receiving the
recognition she felt was her due for her attempts to "live in the
Truth" and lead an environmentally conscious existence. (Both
Natrum muriaticum and *Carcinosin,* torn between a self-isolat-
ing high-mindedness and the desire for worldly approval, have
yet to learn that virtue is its own reward.) First, *Natrum
muriaticum* was administered for her attitude, but helped only
marginally. Then, because there was a history of cancer in the
family, *Carcinosin* was prescribed. Physically, she improved
within a few days and on the mental plane, the remedy helped
lighten her somber outlook on life.

Ralph Waldo Emerson wrote, "God offers to every mind its
choice between truth and repose. Take which you please, you
can never have both." In view of the fact that the young
Carcinosin tends to take life seriously (at times too seriously:
"Today is the tomorrow I agonized over yesterday—and here

I've emerged just fine! Why can't I just take every day as it comes, instead of wasting all that emotional energy worrying about doing right?"), this constitutional type usually opts for the former. Yet it is the remedy's function and part of its benign effect to offer to the overly conscientious or serious child a modicum of repose, even in the worthy pursuit of truth.

❦

Some physical symptoms and characteristics in children that suggest *Carcinosin* are: worms (when a more specific remedy for this condition, like *Cina,* is of no avail); asthma (when *Arsenicum, Nux vomica, Thuja,* or other remedies fail to act); poor sleep; liking of animal fats (*Arsenicum album*) and/or salt (*Natrum muriaticum*); sensitivity to music; a *Sepia*-like marked love of rhythm and dance and liking of thunderstorms; aggravation (*Arsenicum album, Natrum muriaticum*) *or* amelioration (*Natrum muriaticum*) by the seaside; pigmented naevi and moles (*Thuja*); and children who contract a childhood disease more than once or during late adolescence.

Just as the Twig is bent, the Tree's inclined

–Alexander Pope, *Moral Essays, Epistle I*

In the treatment of children, the homoeopathic remedies are renowned for their formative as well as curative role. By administering the constitutional remedy periodically during the different stages of the early formative years, negative emotions or disruptive behavior can be counteracted and a healthy, balanced outlook encouraged. And because the correctly selected similar remedy addresses itself to the unconscious (even more than to the conscious level), homoeopathy is particularly suited to the child who, without needing intellectually to understand his anger, anxieties, or oppositional nature, can relinquish these characteristics. This renders him more free to begin building up the strength and self-confidence required in order to meet constructively the many obstacles and challenges that will confront him (or her) during the process of maturation.

Suggested Readings

The following books will aid the reader in further exploration of homoeopathy; all are currently in print.

Blackie, Margery. *The Patient, Not the Cure.* London: McDonald and Jane's, 1976.

> An excellent overall view of homoeopathy comprising its history, philosophy, *materia medica,* and chronic and acute case illustrations.

Boericke, William. *Materia Medica with Repertory.* New Delhi: B. Jain Publishers, (n.d.)

> An indispensable reference work and learning tool for the aspiring student: the "homoeopathic bible."

Borland, Douglas M. *Children's Types.* London: The British Homoeopathic Association, (n.d.)

> This pioneering work describes in brief some of the lesser as well as the better known children's remedies. Helpful clinical pointers are encountered in its pages.

Coulter, Catherine R. *Portraits of Homoeopathic Medicines: Psychophysical Analyses of Selected Constitutional Types.* Volumes 1-3. Bethesda, Maryland: Ninth House Publishing, 2001 (originally published in 1985 [Vol. 1], 1988 [Vol. 2], and 1998 [Vol. 3]).

> These three volumes explore in depth the interrelations between the mental-emotional and physical symptoms of some

two dozen homoeopathic personality types. *Homoeopathic Sketches of Children's Types* consists, for the most part, of selected passages from this larger work, and extensive bibliographical references and acknowledgments can be found in the three volumes.

_____. *Nature and Human Personality: Homoeopathic Archetypes.* St. Louis: Quality Medical Publishing, 2000.

Twelve *adult* constitutional types, abridged from *Portraits of Homoeopathic Medicines,* vols. 1, 2, and 3.

Panos, Maesimund B., and Heimlich, Jane. *Homoeopathic Medicines at Home.* Los Angeles: JB Tarcher, 1980.

One of the best introductory and self-help books explaining the homoeopathic method and giving indications for prescribing for acute conditions.

Index

Yearling, The; see Rawlings, Marjorie Kinnan
Yielding, 63, 143